Aspects of Social Work and Palliative Care

edited by

Jonathan Parker

Quay Books
MA Healthcare Limited

Quay Books Division, MA Healthcare Limited, St Jude's Church, Dulwich Road,
London SE24 0PB

British Library Cataloguing-in-Publication Data
A catalogue record is available for this book

© MA Healthcare Limited 2005
ISBN 185642 266 6

Printed in the UK by Cromwell Press, Trowbridge, Wiltshire

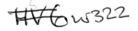

Aspects of Social Work and Palliative Care

Other titles available in the Palliative Care series:

Why is it so difficult to die? by Brian Nyatanga

Fundamental Aspects of Palliative Care Nursing by Robert Becker and Richard Gamlin

Palliative Care for the Child with Malignant Disease edited by The West Midlands Paediatric Team

Palliative Care for the Primary Care Team by Eileen Palmer and John Howarth

Palliative Care for People with Learning Disabilities by Sue Read

Hidden Aspects of Palliative Care by Brian Nyatanga and Maxine Astley-Pepper

Series editor: Brian Nyatanga

Contents

v

Introduction

The care of the sick, the vulnerable and the dying has been a central feature of our history. The provision of care in hospice settings goes back to Islam at the time of the Crusades. It is perhaps not surprising that the highest values of our world's religions find expression in caring for those at the end of life.

Social workers have a particular role to play in this work — a role that is possibly wider than that of other professionals involved. Although social work has a long and illustrious pedigree in hospice work, and attempts at carving out a particular theoretical base and approach have been made by emphasising its 'psychosocial' dimension, it is important not to over-emphasise this dimension or forget that social workers take into account the social needs of the individual in his or her specific life-context. Social work is not only 'holistic' in considering the individual and looking at his or her 'biopsychosocial' and spiritual needs, but it also engages clients' families, friends and other significant people.

But social work's role is wider still. It is 'socio-educative', meaning that social workers in palliative care collaborate with other professionals, volunteers and a wider audience to raise awareness about death, dying and bereavement, and to work towards the reintegration of death and dying into our vision of society.

This book addresses central questions for all social workers, whatever their area of practice and primary service user group and its supporters. Loss, bereavement, grief and mourning are all at the heart of social work's involvement with people.

However, this book delves deeper and more precisely to examine an often neglected area — namely, social work in palliative care settings. Social workers have practised with people who are dying, those who experience potentially life-shortening illnesses, their families and caregivers, for many years. Their role has suffered from lack of attention, and from an over-emphasis on either the practical details of welfare or on the psychological aspects of death, dying and bereavement. How many times have palliative care social workers received requests for assistance filling in benefit forms or for advice concerning charitable awards? How many referrals have been received for 'counselling support', whatever this may mean in practice?

Both welfare support and counselling are important elements of palliative social care work, each emphasised to a lesser or greater degree, depending on setting and team ethos. But this is not the whole story of social work in palliative care. This book addresses some of the dimensions of palliative care and social work that have not gained the attention they deserve, and moves the role of social workers to centre-stage.

It is timely to publish this book as we consolidate social work's image at the beginning of the twenty-first century. Health and social care are high on the Government's agenda for modernising services, joined-up service delivery, and increasing accountability and effective practice. We see this in the production of National Service Frameworks that address health and social care needs in an intertwined way that demands the forging of new ways of working and of the organisation of different disciplines. We must not lose sight of the fact that social workers in palliative care settings have been working in interdisciplinary and multidisciplinary ways since the development of the hospice movement and, indeed, since the inception of hospital almoners in 1895. However, the current emphasis raises new issues: it confirms the importance of working together, but begs questions of management of services; control of delivery; the agendas underpinning such work and its evaluation; and the education needed to carry it out.

The education system for social workers is changing in all four countries within the UK. The standards set for education mean there is a clear opportunity to emphasise palliative care social work and to show just how important it is. Service delivery and its organisation are responding rapidly to the demands for integrated approaches, and service users' and carers' needs are represented and their voices increasingly heard.

This book will be useful for social work students embarking on their professional learning journey. It will provide an insight into palliative care issues and into working with profound loss, grief and mourning. It will also be useful for nursing and medical students and other professions allied to medicine, providing a helpful overview to social work. The book will help other professionals to develop their interprofessional literacy skills, as it will social workers. It is also intended for qualified social workers practising, and working with others, in palliative care settings, and will be of interest to those social workers who perhaps deal only tangentially with death and dying, but come across loss, bereavement and grief in their everyday practice.

It would not be possible to cover all aspects of palliative care social work in a single text. However, this book presents a wide range of central issues in palliative care social work practice and brings together a number of authors with expertise in their particular fields. The authors are social workers from both academic and practice backgrounds, but what unites them all is their passionate commitment to best practice and the highest quality of care in palliative social work settings.

Jonathan Parker
May 2005

Chapter 1

Social work education for palliative care — changes and challenges

Jonathan Parker

Introduction

Social work has a long and varied history. It emerged in Western cultures from the development of urbanisation, industrialism and a search for moral and religious approaches to social problems in a developing secular society, alongside deep-rooted and committed emphases on social justice and political change. In a sense, therefore, it has always focused on those who are displaced; who have experienced loss and need the support of others to (re)join and contribute to the functioning of society. At present, in the UK, dying, death and displays of loss and grief are often shunned, and social work's aim to work alongside those experiencing such phenomena emphasises the connections between palliative care and social work by enfranchising people who have been marginalised by their experiences.

This chapter will briefly chart the development of social work education, placing specific emphasis on learning for working with loss, bereavement and palliative care. As well as examining the generic ways social work programmes might address issues of loss, grief, death and dying, the chapter will focus on specialist programmes that have developed to promote palliative care social work at pre-qualifying and post-qualifying levels. Of course, social work education is concerned with learning in and for practice, as well as with practice in the classroom, and this dual or integrated approach to education will be covered. Social work education is an evolving process and recent changes to qualifying education, and the opportunities this may bring for the inclusion of hospice and palliative care, will be explored.

The development of social work and social work education

Origins

The development of social work practice within the personal social services in the UK is interlinked with corresponding changes and developments in social policy. It is also associated with developments in education and training.

It is possible to trace the development of social welfare in the UK back into history (Horner, 2003). For instance, the Elizabethan Poor Laws of 1598 and 1601 provided relief for the needy of local parishes, laying the foundation for subsequent social security and welfare measures. Also, the eighteenth- and nineteenth-century legislation relating to the care and treatment of people with mental health problems imposed a duty of care and/or control or regulation on local authorities that is echoed in contemporary mental health legislation.

Most commentators, however, chart the development of social work practice in its modern form from one of two points. Douglas and Philpot (1997: 7) suggest that social work:

> *emerged fitfully, from the tide of nineteenth century philanthropy and largely as a voluntary activity, often undertaken by women. Social work is a product of industrialised, urban societies, dealing with the personal consequences of social dislocation.*

Adams (1996) and Sullivan (1996) consider contemporary social work from a more familiar vantage point: the creation and development of the Welfare State in 1948. At whichever point we locate the beginnings of modern social work, it is important to remember, as Pinker (1997) emphasises, that it was the last thirty years of the twentieth century that saw the radical restructuring of the organisation and functioning of statutory and non-statutory social work agencies and professional social work education.

It is important to understand some of the key themes that have underpinned the development of social work. These themes have implications for our understanding of it; the concept of loss, in particular, is central to social work and latterly, by association, to the development of qualifying education. In the nineteenth century, social work was concerned with the relief of poverty and destitution and with the 'rescue' of prostitutes. 'Loss' equated with Christian ideas of being 'lost from God', and social welfare concerned the moral salvation of people brought back into society.

The Victorian era

The roots of this type of social welfare lie in Victorian philanthropy and successive Poor Law legislation. The Poor Law Amendment Act (1834) categorised people as 'deserving' and 'undeserving' poor, which, whatever the distaste evoked by such a distinction, has characterised a recurrent theme throughout the short history of social work. With respect to palliative care and bereavement issues, this dualism reflects those losses that are legitimised and those that are not, and the ways in which people express the felt impact of those losses. For example, in contemporary society, it is likely to be commonly accepted that a person bereaved of their father has a right to grieve openly and might be classed as 'deserving', whereas the death of a distant cousin may not afford such sympathy. The educational issues here are clear: to understand how psychology and culture affect grieving and how attitudes are constructed within society. An approach that seeks to understand meanings and their impact now underpins the values of social work and education, although this has trend has developed over a long period.

To a large extent, the growth of hospice social work is intertwined with medical social work. The development of hospital almoners, arising from the Charitable Organisation Society's (COS) secondment of Miss M Stewart to London's Royal Free Hospital in 1894, was to secure care and assistance for people in need of treatment. But it was the fact that she could detect those who were in a position to pay, but tried to avoid doing so, that captured the imagination of the hospital collecting societies and led to the employment of enquiry agents to prevent fraud. However, developments at the Royal Free led to practical casework training for almoners, under the auspices of the COS, until, in 1907, it was taken over by an independent body, the Hospital Almoners' Council. The emphasis was placed on ability to manage in a practical sense — not on the emotional impact or meaning of loss of health or ability, or loss of loved ones. This focus on practical assistance has characterised hospice social work (Small, 2001) and assessment of practical needs and securing charitable support have formed part of the education for hospice social work from its earliest days.

During the Victorian era, methods and practices developed, including the keeping of systematic records by the Charitable Organisation Society, Ellen Raynard's Bible and Female Mission and the Toynbee Hall Settlement Movement. The facts that were gathered about people were used to make plans and provide help according to perceived needs. This individual approach represented the beginnings of social casework, which, again, has permeated social work's development, reaching its zenith in psychoanalytic approaches (especially in psychiatric social work in the earlier half of the twentieth century) and remaining part of qualifying social work programmes in one guise or another. Indeed, the Department of Health (DoH) (2002) requirements for qualifying social work education stipulate learning about assessment, planning, intervention and review.

The twentieth century

Alongside the religious, moral and philanthropic foundations of social work, there grew, at the turn of the twentieth century, an emphasis on wider social and political factors affecting the welfare and well-being of people. The Settlement Movement and Dr Barnado favoured a group approach to problem-solving and providing assistance at a micro-social level. Beatrice Webb, by contrast, favoured a more radical political response to welfare. She challenged the deterrent effect and stigma of the Poor Law, demanding collective action to achieve minimum conditions in employment and social life. Webb was aided in this by the beginnings of the social survey collected by Charles Booth and Seebohm Rowntree, and a politically reformist approach of government.

The two core emphases of social work education — individual casework (assessment, case planning and intervention) and a growing sense of political and social justice — were established during the fragmented beginnings of social work in the nineteenth century. Throughout the first half of the twentieth century, however, there was no single, formal, social work education programme. Social work itself was inchoate in structure and underpinned by the conflicting discourses of 'deserving/undeserving', casework and radical political action. Some social workers became highly trained, especially psychiatric social workers, but many more remained in voluntary positions in which training and education was minimal (Younghusband, 1981). The gravity of this situation was not ignored and calls for general training mounted (Younghusband, 1951). With the establishment of the Welfare State in 1948, a tripartite system of personal social services — concerning children, physical and mental illness, older and disabled people — was established under local government administration. This system replaced the unwieldy number of independent and Government agencies that provided the range of social services (Sullivan, 1996). This system remained until the early 1970s. But still no unitary system of educating social workers existed.

The post-war years

After the Second World War, a more concerted effort to develop appropriate social work education began, with a call from medical social workers to have at least one university-level course that included a theoretical base in social science, as did existing courses in child care, youth work and family case work. The 1949 Institute of Almoners working party report argued for one-year casework courses to be developed at university level following a general social science course. This led in 1954 to the establishment of a medical social work course at Edinburgh University, followed by others at the London School of Economics (LSE) and the universities of Southampton and Birmingham

(Younghusband, 1978; Pinker, 1997). Towle (1968) called for the inclusion of knowledge and understanding of human behaviour in social work courses. This is central knowledge, alongside the practice approach to funding, finance and care, for social workers working in palliative care settings and, again, comprises a central feature of the requirements for the qualifying degree.

In 1965, the Labour Government established a committee to review local authority social services departments and family services. Whilst the origins of statutory social work had begun with the creation of the welfare state, it is at this point that Adams (1996) claims that modern social work was formally born in England and Wales.

The Seebohm Committee made three recommendations, one of which championed the development of the generic training of social workers and further research into social work practice and welfare. This consolidated the growth in general social work courses that had come to be recognised throughout the 1960s (National Council of Social Service and Women's Employment Federation, 1963), the focus of which was on social science and did not specifically include palliative care, loss, or bereavement work. However, the call for systematic curricula development in social work, and the fact that social workers were expected to work with social and personal difficulties, paved the way to focus on loss in all areas of practice. These recommendations were included in the Local Authority Social Services Act (1970) and generic social services departments were established in 1972.

Seebohm acknowledged that personal problems were often a reflection of wider structural problems in society. As the attitudinal shift took place across departments and agencies providing services, so education shifted its emphasis from personal and family dynamics — casework — to social workers who were capable of carrying out a range of generic tasks; seeing people in their ecological context; and working with the impact of social factors on people's lives. Whether or not the creation of generic social services departments represented Seebohm's intentions accurately (Sullivan, 1996), the social work profession began to train generic as opposed to specialist workers, and this has remained a feature of qualifying social work education since.

Certificate of Qualification in Social Work (CQSW)

Following the implementation of Seebohm, the professional regulatory body for social work at the time, the Central Council for the Education and Training of Social Workers (CCETSW), introduced the Certificate of Qualification in Social Work (CQSW), which set out the content and methods of a course based on generic principles. The CQSW was recognised as the qualifying award for social workers and was regulated and awarded by the professional body, although taught by a range of higher- and further-education institutions. The CQSW included a multidisciplinary knowledge base, using understanding of human growth and behaviour taken from psychology and medicine, as well as social science (Casson, 1982). Social work developed its particular focus on the interplay of interacting systems and how the actions of one may ripple outwards and back inwards to have many evolving implications for all involved (Goldstein, 1973; Pincus and Minahan, 1973; Specht and Vickery, 1977).

The move to generic education and training meant programmes were not specifically focused on one setting or service user group. But the changing emphasis from the individual to the social helped the understanding of the impact of loss and was beneficial, therefore, to palliative care social work. The locus for action grows from the individual, the patient or service user to include consideration of the wider family, friends and 'significant others' in that individual's life. It also allowed social workers to involve wider professional systems and develop practice that is holistic and collaborative. This is something that remains fundamental to contemporary qualifying education for social workers.

Social work practice was reviewed again in the Barclay Report (1982). The Conservative Government of the day was intent on 'rolling back the frontiers of the Welfare State' — that is, reducing dependency on State provision and encouraging family, community and voluntary effort. Social work was seen to be about 'enabling' rather than 'providing'. With the development of contemporary community care policy, social workers became enablers and coordinators rather than providers — care managers who were responsible for the design and purchase of packages of care. These proposals gained all-party backing for a wide variety of disparate reasons and the National Health Service and Community Care Act (1990) was fully implemented in 1993. Whilst the report had little direct impact on social work education, the development of enabling and managing skills permeated skills development.

From DipSW to Social Care Councils

The radical political changes in organisational structure that occurred and the change to a market-dominated purchaser-provider split happened at the same time CCETSW decided to review its training and education. Perhaps this was timely. The Diploma in Social Work (DipSW) was built around a set of rules and competency requirements for the qualification (CCETSW, 1989). Paper 30, as it came to be known, was later revised (CCETSW, 1996). In essence, partnerships between colleges and employing agencies were created to plan course proposals that met the competences and requirements specified for social work education.

Competence in social work education is represented by the integration of knowledge, skills and values. These were reflected in the practice requirements and evidence indicators underpinning the six core competences. Paper 30 continued the generic approach to social work education started with the implementation of Seebohm, but allowed for the development of more specialist teaching, such as palliative care and loss. The knowledge-base for the core competence 'assess and plan' specifically included studying the:

> *social and emotional impact of physical, sensory and learning disabilities, ill health and mental illness in children, adults, families and carers... emotional impact of traumatic events and the range of emotional and psychological reactions to loss, transition and change.*

(CCETSW, 1996: 21)

It was at this time that specialist modules of study, at a qualifying level, were introduced in greater numbers into social work education. The development of competence in communicating with service users, carers and other professionals; coordination of care and support; provision of information and advice; identification of risks; and promotion of a reflective, self-questioning approach — all were open to a wide range of curricula developments.

The professional body, CCETSW, was replaced in 2002 by the creation of Social Care Councils in each of the four UK countries. At the same time, the education and training of social workers was again reviewed. Training and education for qualified social work practice remains within higher education, but the content and methods of training and education are more determined by the demands of practice and the exigencies of social work employers, and those undertaking the qualification.

Contemporary education

Dissatisfaction with the DipSW, expressed by employers of social workers — and as the profession responded to policy shifts and developments; inquiries into cases that had gone tragically wrong; and the need for some level of consistency across qualifications — led to a fundamental review of the training and education of social workers. The result was to develop a new honours degree in social work as the professional qualification for practice. In England, this was implemented in September 2003. Increased emphasis has been placed on practice learning within the new qualifying degree, and the involvement of service users and carers is central.

Until the foundation of the honours degree course, qualifying education for social workers comprised the two-year diploma awarded by the professional body (now the General Social Care Council), which could be delivered and gained in a range of ways, including undergraduate diploma, undergraduate degree plus diploma, postgraduate diploma, or masters degree level. The diploma represented the qualification and was awarded not by the universities and colleges, but by the professional body.

From September 2003 in England, the qualifying award for social work focused on an undergraduate degree delivered and awarded by accredited universities and colleges and approved by the GSCC after university validation of the programme. Wales, Scotland and Northern Ireland introduced their new qualifying programmes in 2004. The core principles for these changes concern the commitment to raising standards, harmonising qualifications and emphasising the centrality of practice learning.

Degree in social work

The degree itself is developed individually within universities, with each institution able to promote its own core areas. However, degrees are built around a complex of regulations, benchmarks and standards, underpinned by values and skills development in extended practice learning settings. They still emphasise the development of competence, exemplified by the integration of values, skills and knowledge.

Subject benchmarks, or specific standards, for honours degrees in social work were developed and published in 2000 (QAA, 2000). These remain the benchmarks for the new qualifying degree, but the new qualification in England also demands integration with National Occupational Standards for social workers (Topss, 2002), DoH Requirements (DoH, 2002), and the Code of Practice for Employees produced by the GSCC (2002). There are also further practical matters to be fulfilled by adherence to GSCC requirements for admission, selection, reporting, delivery and management of the degree. *Figure 1.1* shows the degree's core aspects.

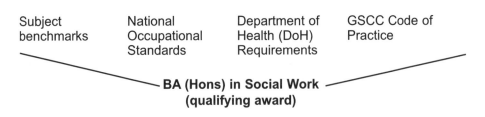

| Subject benchmarks | National Occupational Standards | Department of Health (DoH) Requirements | GSCC Code of Practice |

BA (Hons) in Social Work (qualifying award)

Figure 1.1: Core aspects of the BA (Hons) degree in social work

The structure of the degree has implications for learning and teaching related to palliative care. Although, of course, social work students are not being educated to undertake medical or nursing interventions, some question what it is that social workers are being educated to do. Anecdotal evidence suggests that social workers are seen either as offering counselling support or practical assistance related in particular to the completion of welfare-benefit claims.

Certainly, these activities may comprise a part of the role. There are, however, educative, group and family work, care coordination and management roles taken on by social workers. Often, within the hospice movement, this has been encompassed under the umbrella term of 'psychosocial work' (Sheldon, 1997; Oliviere *et al*, 1998). But although the term may have offered a degree of professional acceptability, it may also have over-emphasised the psychological and intrapersonal (ie. internal-emotional) aspects of the work to the detriment of social and interpersonal (ie. relational) practice. The wider impact that derives from the way society is organised and the ways in which care is delivered, plus the tendency to create particular ways of judging needs, are ignored in this model. Palliative care social work, however, is supported by building on a clear social-science foundation that acknowledges the impact of societal factors on the ways in which loss is perceived and care needs apportioned. Social workers bring a critical perspective that helps balance an over-medicalised approach.

Social work or social security?

People still confuse social services departments and social work with social security. The emphasis on practical assistance in hospice social work (Small, 2001) may have contributed to this confusion. According to Adams (1996), this view reflects the low standing of social work in the minds of the general public. The topic is a difficult one to tackle because of the many conceptions of social work and the lack of consensus on roles, tasks and meaning in social work. Adams (1996: 6) captures this uncertainty well:

> *Social work has a rather weak professional identity partly because social workers deal with a large proportion of the less powerful, less influential and low-status members of society; social workers practise in diverse agencies, roles and settings and, unlike lawyers, doctors and engineers, for example, do not draw upon a body of knowledge and expertise agreed and held in common to all in the profession. There are often uncertainties about what course of action would be most productive and there may be no agreement about this among social workers themselves, let alone among other professionals and... the mass media.'*

The confusion is deepened by the professional and educational distinctions between England, Wales, Scotland and Northern Ireland: these countries have different social work systems and, with the development of the social work degree, each UK administration has developed a separate (albeit transferable) education programme.

It is worth returning to the definition of social work agreed by the IASSW/ IFSW in 2001, which articulates the conjoint activities of intrapersonal and interpersonal work and a commitment to community development and social justice as key to social work in all settings, but which can be developed in palliative care social work in particular.

The themes of social work

The social work profession promotes social change, problem solving in human relationships, and the empowerment and liberation of people to enhance well-being. Utilising theories of human behaviour and social systems, social work intervenes at the points where people interact with their environments. Principles of human rights and social justice are fundamental to social work.

IASSW/IFSW (2001)

Social workers are educated to understand and practise in situations of loss. This is the case when children are separated from their families, and for families that have 'lost' children as a result of social intervention. Social workers work with people experiencing loss as a result of relationship breakdown, redundancy, loss of housing, loss of health, loss of abilities, and so on.

In relation to palliative care and hospice social work, this network of loss still occurs, although it is the loss associated with declining health, limited life expectancy and bereavement that figure most highly in people's minds. These experiences are not singular in effect, and a range of associated losses may figure highly for each individual or family.

Social work education must address loss, theories of loss, grief and bereavement and ways of working with people experiencing loss. This was highlighted by Keating (2002) with respect to social workers practising with bereaved families in Ireland.

Small (2001) acknowledges the significant contribution that UK social work has made to the development of palliative care services, while bemoaning the paucity of literature. There are over two hundred social workers employed in specialist palliative care settings and many more in hospitals, residential and other community settings that work with people at the end stages of life and quite a number in senior positions. Palliative care is recognised as a specialty, having developed from the work of Cicely Saunders and her promotion of hospice as a movement for person-centred care. However, there are still relatively few qualifying programmes that include an overt and significant emphasis on loss and bereavement. These issues are dealt with in the context in which the losses are experienced. This is helpful, but there is room for the development of a more particular focus.

Social work literature dealing with issues of loss, death and dying was sporadically published during the 1940s, 1950s and 1960s (see Clark, 1998). Since 1977, according to Small (2001), a number of themes emerge:

- social work has always been concerned with responding to loss
- social work brings a whole system view, placing the individual in his or her wider ecological context
- social work in palliative care is concerned to deal with the practical as well as emotional, although Lloyd (1997) does suggest that emphasis on the practical must not detract from listening and providing emotional support.

The role of social workers as coordinators and educators, together with their experience of working with volunteers and their knowledge of loss and bereavement, represent important strengths to bring to the palliative care team. The literature also indicates an important role in providing support to the wider multidisciplinary team. Smith (1982) examines the special role social workers have in assisting service users to 'make meaning' from bereavement experiences. Oliviere *et al* (1998) emphasise the focus on the whole person and psychosocial issues. Small (2001: 969) states:

There has been a continuing wish to firmly identify the social work role within palliative care and to argue that it is a role consistent with the overall functions and philosophy of social work… Social work, as undertaken within the palliative care team, has looked to the emerging practice and the established principles of hospice and palliative care. It has less often reflected the strains and achievements of the broader social work community. The values of social work and palliative care are linked.

In working in palliative care settings, there is a further need to develop a wide professional and interprofessional literacy. Social workers do not work in a vacuum, and if they are to play a full part in palliative care settings, they need an understanding of hospice, health and social care service delivery; social and health care policies with people who are dying or have a life-threatening illness; and an understanding, at theoretical and practical levels, of the roles and tasks associated with other professions working within that context. Continuing professional development and education is warranted here.

Education programmes

There is a great deal of emphasis on education for palliative care: often, it is non-qualifying and/or health professional-focused, such as the Scottish Partnership for Palliative Care (SPPC; www.palliativecarescotland.org.uk) and Douglas' (2002) in-house work on bereavement education for nurses or support staff (Brown, Burns and Flynn, 2003). Nurse education for palliative care is innovative and well-supported. For instance, van Boxel *et al* (2003) report a study into the effectiveness of face-to-face and video-conferenced teaching delivery to community nurses. The study found that both were equally effective in promoting learning, thereby opening up possibilities for reaching a greater number of professionals. Kenny (2003) uses thinking games to encourage critical and reflective practice in nurses in palliative care.

Palliative education is also developing within medical education, showing an increasing emphasis within the curriculum on symptom relief, attitudes to death and dying, and sometimes using the dying patient as instructor (Field and Wee, 2002). The usefulness of such programmes is not in doubt (Ferrell and Borneman, 2002), but many also recognise that improvements in palliative care education for health professionals are needed (Reb, 2003; Piller, 2001).

Post-qualifying programmes

There are an increasing number of post-qualifying programmes that are offered on a multiprofessional basis. There is also a growing emphasis on undergraduate interprofessional teaching (Wee *et al*, 2001; Weinstein, 2002), although there is a lack so far of rigorous evaluation of learning in these innovations (Barr, 2002). The value of interprofessional learning and the ability to deal with distressing situations by undergraduate students is clear, as is the importance and potential catharsis for carers contributing to these programmes (Turner *et al*, 2000; Turner, 2001; Latimer *et al*, 1999).

This is an important factor, as it is now imperative for social work students to learn about collaborative ways of practising, and interprofessional education is seen as fundamental in health and social care. The DoH (2002) consider working together across professions to be a requirement of qualifying programmes. Palliative care and hospice social work and issues provide a useful focus to develop such understanding. This is especially the case in developing practice learning opportunities for social work students.

The inclusion of palliative care as a core uniprofessional feature of qualifying programmes has been minimal. The degree offers a chance to rectify this, although programme planners may be put off from doing so because of the tight timescales set for delivery of an intensive programme and the increased demands for practice learning. Opportunities involved in developing interprofessional approaches with health-related students offer a way forward and meet a core component of the DoH's (2002) requirements for social work education. The emphasis on statutory working in the degree must not detract from the evolution of creative approaches to joint learning in voluntary and charitable body settings, especially with respect to practice learning opportunities. Programmes can begin to seize the momentum for constructive educational development by acknowledging the centrality of issues of loss, working to the new health and social care agenda and increasing interprofessional opportunities.

The teaching of palliative care

The teaching of palliative care to social work students studying at undergraduate and postgraduate levels for a DipSW at the University of Hull began in 1993 with the appointment of a Macmillan Lecturer in Palliative Care Social Work — one of a handful appointed at the time. In early years, the focus was enhanced by teaching that was specifically related to HIV and AIDS, although latterly it is hospice, palliative care, loss and bereavement that is emphasised within the curriculum. Palliative care and social work developed as a specialist pathway on the programme, attracting students on a national basis because of the palliative care focus. The teaching developed at this time covered such topics as:

- the hospice movement and history of palliative care
- theories of bereavement, health and illness
- health and social care policy related to palliative care
- visiting local palliative care agencies and funeral directors
- dealing with death and dying
- understanding death
- working with loss in a range of areas and situations.

The teaching was modular, representing a focused area of study that relates to social work with adults, children and families, but is linked to the programme as a whole meeting the requirements for social work qualifying awards. Originally, there were five aims to the programme, including:

- ❖ Providing a theoretical framework for understanding the processes of loss and grief.
- ❖ Examining ways in which this framework can help social workers understand personal and social changes and losses, and their effects on individuals and families.
- ❖ Looking at the meanings of loss and change with people who are dying, bereaved, sensory-impaired, facing loss by separation or as a result of substance use.

- ❖ Focusing in particular on palliative care and losses experienced by those facing life-threatening illnesses and those around them.
- ❖ Considering bereavement work as an integral part of palliative care social work.

The teaching progressed in stages — considering the theoretical underpinnings to understanding loss, bereavement, palliative care and its history — while also beginning to examine personal feelings about loss. The learning process was enhanced by students working in small groups to develop presentations concerning working with loss and bereavement in the final week of the course. The opportunity to examine some of the processes involved in working with people who are dying and significant people around them was developed through case study work, discussion and meeting with practitioners in the area. Students visit a local hospice and locate the position of social workers in palliative care within a multidisciplinary setting, considering their specific roles and functions. They also have the opportunity to visit a funeral director's premises, dispelling many of the myths held by students about what happens to the dead, and also stressing the importance of the funeral as a rite in the human experience of death and bereavement.

This 'experiential' approach to teaching and learning accords with adult learning principles in which students identify their starting point, their preferred methods of learning, then engage in a range of pedagogical activities to develop understanding. Students report a high degree of participation in the programme, especially with respect to the development and presentation of their own workshop on loss and bereavement.

However, the opportunity to discuss their own experiences is also appreciated. As one student said, 'relating personal experiences of loss was useful'. Another student commented, 'I liked the way that death, grief and bereavement were "normalised". It was interesting, informative and relevant'. The teaching began as an introduction to social work in palliative care, but, over the years, it has included a greater focus on issues of loss and bereavement as central to the social work role, and knowledge that is transferable across social work roles and functions.

The revised degree in social work

In the revised qualifying social work degree, the aims and intended learning outcomes have been adjusted slightly to reflect the changes to (and widening of) the requirements for social work education. The aims are simpler and centre on theories of loss, grief and bereavement; the effects on individuals and families; and how palliative care and bereavement services can assist people.

The success that the module has enjoyed — in terms of student feedback, the national profile of the programme, and in students securing specialist palliative care posts — has reinvigorated the team to continue a palliative care and hospice focus. The action-focused and experiential approach remains in place and is supplemented by an emphasis on sharing personal and professional experiences and developing presentation material. Students do receive a 'health warning' before taking this module because of the nature of the work. However, experience has taught us that a great deal of learning, albeit painful at times, can result form explore raw and personal experiences.

As *Table 1.1* shows, palliative care and bereavement teaching meets the core requirements of the DoH.

Table 1.1: Palliative care and bereavement teaching		
Macro level	**Mezzo level**	**Micro level**
The social and political realm	*Knowledge and value bases*	*Practice skills*
Inter-professional working, legislation	Understanding human growth and development; context, values and cultural	Communication skills; processes of assessment, planning, intervention and review

It could be argued that the degree requirements make it more likely that other social work qualifying programmes will focus more specifically on issues of loss, grief, bereavement and palliative care because of the core areas — in particular, communication, inter-professional working, human growth and development, disability and mental health — and because of the common experience of loss in its many forms across all fields and disciplines in social work. We shall have to wait and see. The higher education criteria for social work degrees, known as subject benchmarking criteria (QAA, 2000), also emphasise developing and demonstrating communication skills, a broad level of social work knowledge and interprofessional working, and the National Occupational Standards for Social Work (Topss, 2002) promote competence in working with and supporting people. The combination of these generic requirements can be met in a range of ways.

However, teaching palliative care, bereavement and loss lies at the heart of social work and produces knowledge, skills and a value-base that can be transferred across the many settings in which social workers practise. All social workers work with and experience loss and grief. Whether working with children and families (or more specialist adoption settings); with people with mental health problems; people with disabilities; older people; or in hospital and specialist palliative care teams, anticipated, sudden, progressive and protracted experiences of loss will be encountered. By explicitly focusing on loss, bereavement and palliative care issues, programme providers may find a way of developing the skills and knowledge to be effective, while also promoting skills and values within practitioners to deal safely with strong emotions and to look after themselves.

Ethical issues surrounding euthanasia

Leichtentritt (2002) has called for the ethical issues surrounding euthanasia in social work to be included in education and training. This call stems from his research into attitudes to 'active' and 'passive' euthanasia among Israeli social workers. ('Active' euthanasia denotes assistance given to the person to hasten death, whereas 'passive' euthanasia denotes taking no action to prolong life or to prevent death.) Leichtentritt writes:

> *Until professional guidelines are widely available around the world,*
> *social workers ought to at least examine their own meanings and*
> *attitudes towards the universal phenomenon of euthanasia. The*
> *subject needs to be included in professional training programmes*
> *and socialisation processes. The social work profession cannot allow*
> *itself to ignore this issue; ignorance and a lack of discourse are the*
> *most dangerous forms of addressing and practising euthanasia.*

(Leichtentritt, 2002: 411)

At the University of Hull, UK, the ethics of euthanasia are central to palliative care education. Education for social work practice was improved by the development of a constructive partnership between the University of Hull and the local hospice social work team. Palliative care teaching has been developed in such a way as to be co-delivered, which ensures that practice and theory are fully integrated; that successful students pursuing this module are 'fit for practice and purpose'; and that learning is seen as an essential criterion of continually improving practice.

The importance of including service users in planning and improving services is paramount to contemporary health and socials care. It is also part of the requirements for social work education. One area in which we are exploring links is the involvement of service-user groups and individuals who offer significant insights into service and education requirements. Where these can be combined, and service users want it to happen, attention will be given to improving the teaching and learning partnership to bring it about.

Not only is the palliative care programme taught by the hospice/university partnership, but practice learning opportunities are also given a high priority. In the degree course, students must have experience of statutory social work, including legal interventions (DoH, 2002). This has caused some consternation in the development of the Hull model for partner practitioners who rightly point out that social workers are increasingly employed outside the statutory sector and within health care settings in which traditionally defined statutory work may not be undertaken.

However, the increasing emphasis on multiprofessional responses to health and social care issues adds an important policy perspective and developing opportunities for experiencing statutory-required tasks. In order to meet these stipulations, collaboration is being developed between the local hospice and local authority statutory partners to create practice learning experiences that include community care assessments and will incorporate the single assessment process locally.

The location of social work within university settings offers opportunities for the future development of palliative care teaching. The Social Work Department forms part of the Faculty of Health and Social Care, including nurse education, health promotion and links with the Hull-York Medical School. This scenario provides an opportunity to develop a multiprofessional and shared learning perspective that will meet the current agenda and help in promoting learning about loss, bereavement, grief and palliative care, as well as an understanding of the roles of different professionals working in this area.

References

Adams R (1996) *The Personal Social Services*. Longman, Harlow

Barclay P (1982) *Social Workers: their Roles and Tasks*. The report of a working party set up in October 1980 at the request of the Secretary of State for Social Services by the National Institute for Social Work under the chairmanship of Mr Peter M. Barclay. Bedford Square Press, London

Barr H (2002) *Interprofessional Education Today, Yesterday and Tomorrow: Occasional Paper No. 1*. Learning and Teaching Support Network, London

Brown H, Burns S, Flynn M (2003) Please don't let it happen on my shift: supporting staff who are caring for people with learning disabilities who are dying. *Tizard Learn Disabil Rev* **8**(2): 32–41

Casson P (1982) *Social Work Courses: their Structure and Content*. CCETSW, London

CCETSW (1991) *Rules and Requirements for the Diploma in Social Work*. CCETSW, London

CCETSW (1996) *Assuring Quality in the Diploma in Social Work: 1. Rules and Requirements for the DipSW*. 2nd edition/2nd revision. CCETSW, London

Clark D (1998) An annotated bibliography of the publications of Cicely Saunders — 1, 1958–67. *Palliat Med* **12**(3): 181–93

DoH (2002) *Requirements for Social Work Training*. DoH, London

Douglas M (2002) Addressing bereavement issues through education. *Nurs Times* **15 October 2002**: 36–7

Douglas A, Philpot T (1997) *Caring and Coping: a Guide to Social Services.* Routledge, London

Ferrell B, Borneman T (2002) Community implementation of home care palliative care education. *Cancer Pract* **10**(1): 20–7

Field D, Wee B (2002) Preparation for palliative care: teaching about death, dying and bereavement in UK medical schools 2000–2001. *Med Educ* **36**(6): 561–7

Goldstein H (1973) *Social Work Practice: a Unitary Approach.* University of South Carolina Press, Columbia, South Carolina

GSCC (2002) *Codes of Practice for Social Care Workers and Employers.* GSCC, London

Horner N (2003) *What is Social Work?* Learning Matters, Exeter

Keating A (2002) Impending loss to bereavement after care: a medical social work approach. *Ir Soc Worker* **20**(3/4): 30–2

Kenny L (2003) Using Edward de Bono's six hats game to aid critical thinking and reflection in palliative care. *Int J Palliat Nurs* **9**(3): 105–12

Latimer E, Deakin A, Ingram C, O'Brien L, Smoke M, Wishart L (1999) An interdisciplinary approach to a day-long palliative care course for undergraduate students. *Can Med Assoc J* **161**(6): 729–31

Leichtentritt R (2002) Euthanasia: Israeli social workers' experiences, attitudes and meanings. *Br J Soc Work* **32**(4): 397–413

Lloyd M (1997) Dying and bereavement, spirituality and social work in a market economy of welfare. *Br J Soc Work* **27**: 175–90

Oliviere D, Hargreaves R, Monroe B (1998) *Good Practice in Palliative Care.* Ashgate, Aldershot

Piller N (2001) Provider perspectives on palliative care needs at a major teaching hospital. *Palliat Med* **15**(6): 461–70

Pincus A, Minahan A (1973) *Social Work Practice: Model and Method Hasca.* Peacock, Illinois

Pinker R (1997) Recent trends in British social policy and their implications for social work practice and education. *Issues Soc Work Educ* **17**(2): 31–47

QAA (2000) *Subject Benchmark Statements: Social Policy and Administration and Social Work.* QAA, Gloucester

Reb A (2003) Palliative and end-of-life care: policy analysis. *Oncol Nurs Forum* **30**(1): 35–50

Sheldon F (1997) *Psychosocial Palliative Care: Good Practice in the Care of the Dying and Bereaved.* Stanley Thomas, Cheltenham

Smith C (1982) *Social Work with the Dying and the Bereaved.* Macmillan, London

Specht H, Vickery A (1977) *Integrating Social Work Methods.* Allen and Unwin, London

Small N (2001) Social work and palliative care. *Br J Soc Work* **31**(6): 961–71

Sullivan M (1996) *The Development of the British Welfare State.* Prentice-Hall/Harvester Wheatsheaf, Hemel Hemspstead

Topss (2002) *National Occupational Standards for Social Work.* Topss England, London

Towle C (1968) The place of help in supervision. In: Younghusband E (ed) *Education for Social Work: Readings in Social Work Vol IV*. NISW, London

Turner P (2001) Palliative care: a suitable setting for undergraduate interprofessional education. *Palliat Med* **15**(1): 487–92

Turner P, Sheldon F, Coles C, Mountford B, Hillier R, Radway P, Wee B (2000) Listening to and learning from the family carer's story: an innovative approach in interprofessional education. *J Interprof Care* **14**(4): 387–95

Van Boxel P, Anderson K, Regnard C (2003) The effectiveness of palliative care education delivered by video-conferencing compared with face-to-face delivery. *Palliat Med* **17**(4): 344–59

Wee B, Hiller R, Coles C, Mountford B, Sheldon F, Turner P (2001) Palliative care: a suitable setting for undergraduate interprofessional education. *Palliat Med* **15**: 487–92

Weinstein J (2002) Teaching and learning about loss. In: Thompson N (ed) *Loss and Grief: a Guide for Human Service Practitioners*. Palgrave, Basingstoke

Younghusband E (1951) *Social Work in Britain: a Supplementary Report on the Employment and Training of Social Workers*. T & A Constable, Edinburgh

Younghusband E (1978) *Social Work in Britain: 1950–1975*. George Allen and Unwin, London

Younghusband E (1981) *The Newest Profession: a Short History of Social Work*. IPC, Sutton

Chapter 2

What service users want from specialist palliative care social work — findings from a participatory research project

Suzy Croft, Peter Beresford, Lesley Adshead

Background

Involving patients or service users in palliative care and palliative care research raises its own complex, practical, methodological and ethical issues. Generally, so far, there has been relatively little attempt to involve palliative care service users in research and evaluation. But that omission raises its own ethical and methodological issues. It flies in the face of increasing current pressures to involve patients, public and service users in research and evaluation, as well as in policy and practice. It also imposes an arbitrary limit on the knowledge-base of palliative care policy and practice and on the ways in which that knowledge is collected and developed. The Involve! project was an attempt to take forward user involvement in this complex area of research. In this chapter, we will explore how we undertook the research and some of its key findings.

Introduction to the project

The Involve! project was a three-year national research project, supported by the Joseph Rowntree Foundation. It gained its name before the Government NHS Research and Development body — Consumers in NHS Research, which was commissioned to increase public and user involvement in research — changed its name to Involve! The project set out to explore what service users wanted from specialist palliative care social work. Its focus was service users' perspectives on such social work, to establish what it was like for them, what they thought of it, and what ideas they had about it. It was concerned with both the process and the outcomes of practice for service users and with developing user-defined outcome measures. In this sense, it can be seen as relating to the 'quality' debate about health and social care, but coming from a different standpoint to the dominant discussion.

The project included the range of settings for such social work, including independent hospices, NHS hospice units, hospital oncology units, and palliative care day centres. It distinguished between two groups of service users and included both: those who were living with a life-threatening illness or condition, and those who had been bereaved. The research sought to find out through in-depth, qualitative methods the observations and views of both these groups. People were interviewed either as individuals or through group discussions, using a semi-structured schedule.

A total of 111 people were interviewed in the project. Sixty-one were bereaved and fifty-two had life-limiting illnesses and conditions (two people were both bereaved and patients). Seventy-two people were interviewed individually and there were seven group discussions, including a total of thirty-nine people. The project included thirty-nine men and seventy-three women. Nine perc ent of participants identified themselves as black and/or members of minority ethnic groups. Service users came from twenty-six different specialist palliative care settings, located in urban, suburban, rural, small-town and coastal settings in England, Scotland, Wales and Northern Ireland.

The aim of the project was to provide an opportunity for service users to identify what actually happens in specialist palliative care social work; their definitions of the key issues; their views about good practice; what works and what doesn't; and what outcomes they desire from their involvement with specialist palliative care social work. Based on this, the overall aim was to inform the knowledge-base of palliative care social work, to develop policy and practice, and to improve training and education.

The research used a participatory approach and service users were involved in both the design and management of the project. We aimed to involve specialist palliative care service users in all stages of the project.

Service users were included in the advisory group, which the Joseph Rowntree Foundation generally requires their projects to have. This group met eight times throughout the life of the project and included two users of specialist palliative care services (people with life-limiting conditions), as well as other social care service users. We also set up three steering groups of palliative care social work service users to meet throughout the project and produced newsletters to keep everyone we interviewed, whether as individuals or as groups, informed and involved in the progress of the work. Clearly, what we are discussing in this chapter is an example of user involvement in research, rather than user-controlled research.

Ethical issues around involving service users

Involving service users in palliative care research raises its own particular ethical issues and challenges. When we undertook this project, we had to be sure that it was right to talk to people who might be extremely ill. We know that some people died not long after we interviewed them. There are also ethical issues around involving in research bereaved people who may be very vulnerable as they undergo the emotional upheavals and the practical difficulties that often follow bereavement. The project was granted formal ethical approval, but many more ethical issues needed to be addressed.

Two of us had previously been involved in setting up a national seminar on user involvement in palliative care which was held at St Christopher's hospice in London in July, 1999. The seminar was planned and organised by a group of service users and professionals in the fields of palliative care and user involvement. About seventy people, mainly service users, attended that seminar and said very clearly that they wanted to be involved and were prepared to give up time and energy so that services could be improved, if not for themselves, then at least for future service users (Beresford *et al*, 2000).

The seminar showed clearly that people who are very ill can be involved effectively, if suitable support is put in place and the event is structured appropriately and sensitively. Our starting point was, therefore, that it was not just appropriate but also important to involve users of palliative care services in this type of research and this was borne out by what was later expressed in the steering groups. We also thought through the ethical implications of a number of related issues. These included the following categories.

Recruitment

We decided to use specialist palliative care social workers to help us find service users to interview. We wanted to be sure that service users were not at a stage in their illness or bereavement where it would be inappropriate and unhelpful to involve them. This meant that social workers would not approach anyone who was experiencing extreme distress or who might already have been asked to take part in other research projects, as we did not want to overload people.

Information needs

We were aware that some service users might feel obliged to take part if asked by a social worker to whom they felt particularly grateful, so we provided an information sheet for all participants which described the project and its aims.

It also made clear that their involvement was entirely voluntary and that they could withdraw at any time without explanation.

The information sheet provided a contact name and address so service users could phone and ask for information should they wish. It was also made clear that they could do this after an interview if they wanted to ask questions, make further comments or criticisms, or if they needed support. The information sheet emphasised that the project was independent of the service they used and any workers working with them. It avoided terms such as 'terminal illness' and 'dying', as we knew that some participants preferred not to address or refer to that part of their illness or condition, or to refer to it in that way.

Confidentiality and consent

Our information sheet made it clear that information would not be fed back to the social worker unless the participant expressly requested this. It also stated that no participant would be identified by name in future publications. We highlighted the emphasis we placed on confidentiality.

The interviews

The interview schedule was deliberately drafted so as to avoid having to ask intrusive or searching questions. We did not ask anyone about the nature of their illness or condition, but rather invited the service user to tell their story about their involvement with palliative care and palliative care social work in their own words. We used a semi-structured interview schedule, which service users were involved in designing, which included a high proportion of open-ended questions. In this way, we hoped that control over the interview lay with the service user, as far as was possible. As we recognised that some service users might want to talk about painful and difficult experiences, all the interviews were carried out by people either with experience as specialist palliative care social workers themselves, or by others with similar training and backgrounds. Interviewees were told that they could stop and rest at any time, or stop the interview altogether if they wished.

It was vital to us that service users could use the interview to talk at length and in detail about what was important to them without the interviewer becoming too prescriptive. We encouraged participants to 'take off' in directions of their own choosing in interviews and group discussions. Interviewing and facilitation required particular skill to maintain a balance between our need to address certain questions, and opportunities for service users to retain control of the process.

Meeting people's support needs

For all the groups and individuals who took part, we tried to ensure that their involvement in the project was as comfortable as possible and that any costs of taking part, whether financial, emotional, practical or physical, were minimal. We interviewed people at their own choice of venue, offered refreshments and met the costs of travel and other expenses.

A further reason for recruiting participants through the specialist palliative care social workers was that we knew that the social worker would be on hand to offer extra support after an interview, should someone feel they needed it. We gave contact details so that participants could get back in touch with us if they wanted. We could also offer professional palliative care support skills, but the availability of social workers represented an additional and ongoing resource.

One social worker commented that the whole process had been quite a learning experience for her. She felt that some of the people interviewed had needed 'a bit of nurturing afterwards' as, for example, in one case, when the interviewee's bereavement 'came flooding back'. Another social worker asked us to be aware, before we interviewed two women she had been working with, that they both felt they had been 'healed by God'. She rightly wanted to make sure the interviewer would be especially sensitive to the fact that not everyone can or does talk about dying when they are very ill.

We also wrote a card to each participant after an interview or group discussion, giving a name and number and making clear we were available to be contacted. In fact, one participant wrote to the person who had interviewed her to let her know of some good news she had had about her illness and treatment.

Feedback and further involvement

It was seen as very important to let the service users who participated in the project know what we had learned from them and to know how this information might be used in the future. This was done through the newsletter, mentioned above, which was distributed to service users who were interviewed and to members of the steering groups.

The steering groups

One of the ways we sought to ensure that palliative care service users would have an effective and continuing role in influencing and guiding the project was through establishing a series of 'steering groups'.

Initially, three steering groups were established. Two were made up of a mixture of service users facing life-limiting illnesses and conditions, and people who had been bereaved. One consisted only of patients. The steering groups were set up in three different locations: a voluntary hospice in a deprived inner city area of a large city; a voluntary hospice in a rural area; and a voluntary hospice for people living with HIV/AIDS on the south coast. In two of the hospices, we enlisted the help of the social worker in setting up the group. In the hospice for people with HIV/AIDS, the group was brought together by the chair of the clients' forum at that hospice, who was himself a service user.

The aim was for the steering groups to meet about four times throughout the project. We recognised that many people might die during the project and our aim was to ensure some continuity of involvement for the steering groups, even though their membership might change. In the event, one of the groups met twice and the other two groups only once, but we went on to have a steering group meeting with a group of patients in a voluntary day hospice in the Midlands, who had previously been interviewed as part of the research.

We asked the steering groups about their views and experiences of palliative care social work and for their suggestions as to how the project should go about getting the views of other service users. We also asked for their feedback on how the work was progressing. For example, at the first meeting, we asked for comments and feedback on the draft interview schedule we had drawn up for individual interviews and group discussions.

We produced information for the steering groups to be given out to each person attending beforehand. This leaflet provided a contact name and address, so that if people had any further comments or worries, or felt upset about anything, they could contact the named person after the meeting. We also wrote to everyone who came to each meeting, thanking them for taking part and again giving a contact name and address. One steering group member did subsequently contact us in this way. Any travelling or other expenses were paid.

Issues for user involvement raised by the steering groups

Incorporating service users into the steering groups raised a number of significant issues in relation to developing supportive and ethical user involvement.

It quickly became clear that the service users who took part in the steering groups were very interested in the project and genuinely wanted to offer comments and suggestions. Several people said how good it felt to be involved and to be able to offer some of their 'expertise' and not just to be defined as a 'patient'. We were struck by how anxious people were to continue their involvement and how much they emphasised they wanted to be kept in touch. One woman who was moving to Scotland to be nearer her family, asked to be kept abreast of what happened. We had no sense of people wanting to rush off or of feeling the whole exercise was peripheral or a waste of time.

The members of the steering group from the hospice in the Midlands, who had previously been interviewed as part of a patient group, said how pleased they were to know what was happening with the project and to have a chance to be involved again. Apart from one woman who was too ill to attend, all of those who took part in the first discussion, held as part of the research, came to the steering group meeting.

Although a lot of painful issues were raised by and for people, the steering groups seemed to 'gel' very quickly. However, a crucial ethical issue related to mixing people with life-limiting conditions and bereaved people was raised by one group member, a man facing a terminal illness. He contacted our worker after the first meeting and said that he knew he was dying from his brain tumour and welcomed the opportunity to talk about it in the group. He also valued the support he was receiving from the specialist palliative care social worker. But he was concerned that the bereaved people in the group might be upset if, for example, they related his experiences to the loved one who had died.

This was a very important point. The facilitators had noticed that during the discussion, one woman who had been bereaved did seem to find it more upsetting than other group members. She said she found it very difficult to talk and did not stay on for lunch. In the event, we were unable to meet again with this particular group, but if we had, we would have had to address this issue beforehand with group members, and it may have been appropriate to meet with bereaved people and people with life-limiting illnesses as two separate groups.

The steering groups were an essential part of the project and were basically 'business' meetings which had an important agenda in terms of the research. People knew this when they came and were happy to focus on the research project, but we recognised it was also very important to be respectful of the personal experiences and accounts that participants had to tell. In groups like these, it takes quite a while for introductions to be made, for people to settle down with a cup of tea and feel comfortable. Often, those taking part were raising painful and difficult issues. It was not always easy or appropriate to move people on from 'telling their story' or when they were talking about the idea of their own death. In the event, a lot of helpful and useful work was done and, judging by the feedback, people enjoyed participating.

Another issue we encountered in terms of service user involvement was that of gatekeeping. In one hospice, although the social worker was willing to help, the hospice management insisted that until it had been cleared by the ethics committee, we could not invite service users to take part in the steering group. Yet of course we were not seeking to involve them as research 'participants' but in a co-researcher role. People imbued with traditional understandings of research and research relationships (and the role of the service user/patient within them) seem to find this distinction difficult to recognise. The social worker had to make a presentation to the ethics committee on our behalf using the material we sent her — and this overcame objections.

We also encountered difficulties setting up a second meeting of the steering group at this and another hospice. We were reliant on the continuing help of social workers to use their facilities and to let us know if any of the service users who had been involved in the first steering group had subsequently died, so that we did not send out letters that could cause distress to their family or friends. In the event, we did not hear back from one of the two hospices, while the social worker at the other made clear that the situation there was currently 'difficult' owing to 'reorganisation'. We do not know if the lack of response from the first hospice was because of other pressing priorities or organisational changes. Nor were we subsequently able to revisit these hospices, although we were able to maintain positive relationships with staff involved.

By contrast, it was remarkably easy to arrange a second meeting at the hospice for people living with HIV/AIDS. Our original (service user) contact had moved on, but there was no difficulty in setting up the group again, which included some of the original members. We wondered if this is because, being a centre for people with HIV/AIDS which had its own clients' forum, it has a much more developed philosophy of treating clients/patients as equals — that is, as people who have a right to know what they are being asked and the choice of saying 'yes' or 'no' for themselves.

Findings from the project

A key aim of the Involve! project was to identify what service users wanted from specialist palliative care social work and what outcomes they particularly valued. This objective relates to broader work that has been developed by the independent national user controlled organisation, Shaping Our Lives, which has been exploring outcome measures for health and social care since 1996. Shaping Our Lives, which is core funded by the Department of Health (DoH) and receives support from the Joseph Rowntree Foundation, has sought to develop work with service users on user-defined outcome measures to add to the managerial and professional measures that have so far tended to predominate (Balloch *et al*, 1998; Beresford *et al*, 1997; Schalock, 1995; Shaping Our Lives National User Network *et al*, 2003; Turner, 1997, 1998). What service users want from workers and services may not be the same as what service providers and agencies want (Harding and Beresford, 1996).

In the work that Shaping Our Lives has done, two issues have repeatedly emerged. First, the outcomes for service users cannot be separated from the process of services and occupational practice. People are unlikely to experience a positive outcome from a negative process. Second, while each individual service user may prioritise different personal outcomes and want different things from practitioners and services, there do seem to be common themes. For example, to be treated with equality and respect, and for their human and civil rights to be recognised and safeguarded.

The findings of the Involve! project reinforce the broad idea that it is neither helpful nor possible to separate the process of practice from its outcomes for service users. Key outcomes for service users seem to centre on having adequate and appropriate support to deal with both the practical issues that may face people experiencing bereavement and life-limiting conditions, and also the psychological and emotional issues. Almost all participants in the project expressed very positive views of the specialist palliative care social workers working with them. Participants in the project highlighted a number of qualities and skills which they felt enabled specialist palliative care social workers to offer such support. These include the following.

A positive relationship

The relationship between the specialist palliative care social worker and the patient/bereaved person emerged as central. This was emphasised repeatedly by participants in the project. What they particularly valued was the sense that the social worker was treating them with respect as a human being. Some service users commented that the relationship felt like a friendship, albeit one with clear professional limits. They spoke of the social worker as someone who cared, sometimes in place of family if there was no family, or if family life was difficult. They said that the social worker helped them feel in control. One man said the social worker literally 'saved my life', because she helped him overcome the suicidal feelings he had been experiencing. For example:

> *She's genuine. Honestly, I think she genuinely cares about you.*
>
> (white UK male patient, age group 46–55 years)

> *I was looking forward to her coming as a friend. I felt I could talk to her about anything. I wouldn't need to watch my tongue… I had complete confidence in her.*
>
> (white UK bereaved woman, age group 75 years and over)

Listening to service users

Service users reported that they felt the social worker had been prepared to listen to them and had thus felt very involved in the process of working out what needed to be done and what issues were important to them. For instance:

> *She was just prepared to listen. She listened, basically, and where she felt she needed to give some counselling, advice, whatever, she would offer it to me, but she wouldn't force it on me.*
>
> (black UK female patient, age group 26–35 years)

> *She was just there to listen to me and I was the one that did most of the talking and I kind of led the actual meeting...*
>
> (white UK female patient, age group 56–65 years)

Seeing 'the person'

Knowing the 'real person' as opposed to the 'patient' also seemed to be a key positive factor for service users. Only by knowing the real person can the social worker be an effective advocate and establish trust. It was very important for bereaved people, too, that the social worker had seen the process of the illness and the changes it had wrought. The social worker had come to know 'the full story', good and bad.

> [The social worker] *definitely saw me as a person and saw, I think, probably that I was not the person I used to be.*
>
> (a patient taking part in a group discussion)

Having time

Practitioners 'having time' was seen as vitally important by the people we interviewed. Specialist palliative care social workers contrasted positively with other professionals, including other social workers, particularly local authority care managers. The knowledge and sense that the social worker had time enabled fuller discussion and a chance to get to know each other. Many people commented positively that they felt they had got to know the social worker well. In this way, the relationship contained an element of reciprocity that was highly valued. For example:

> *I can't emphasise the time scale of things. There's no rush, you don't feel you are being a burden or that you know you are wasting their time somehow. You know she's always got the time you need.*
>
> (a white widowed UK mother of three young children, age group 26–35 years)

The range of help available

People also commented on how much they valued the range of help that was available from many specialist palliative care social workers. This included help with benefits, access to housing, support for their family and friends, access to a group to meet others in a similar situation through to individual counselling, which often went on for as long as that person needed it. It also became apparent that the same social worker would offer different forms of support to different people according to what they wanted.

> *I know that if there is anything that is worrying me or I need to know or ask, I can ask her and if she doesn't know she will know who to ask.*
>
> (white UK male patient, age group 26–35 years)

Competent workers

Specialist palliative care social workers were seen as experienced, knowledgeable and skilful. They were also prepared to get involved in a very 'hands on' way and this seemed to help service users feel in control. It gave them a belief that they could cope. They knew that at their next meeting with the social worker, they could raise their anxieties with them.

> *She not only understands the patient and the partner of the patient, she understands the systems as well… It's obvious to us that she knows her job inside out.*
>
> (husband of a white UK female patient, age group 56–65 years)

The informality of referral

Service users valued the informal way in which most of them had been approached by the social worker. Several said they had been approached without any formal request or referral, and many told us they appreciated this kind of approach, which made them feel safe and cared for. Most social workers were clearly not using formal referrals, agendas or checklists.

But this did not mean that practitioners were working on a 'hit or miss' basis; rather, they were avoiding the more mechanistic approaches to referral that have developed more generally in social work, particularly in the field of care management. This worked well where people may have had negative views about social workers in general (see below), leading them to reject more formal approaches. Some of the men, in particular, said they liked the fact that they had not been given too much choice, and that the social worker had turned up uninvited. They agreed that given the choice, they might have refused the support which they later found helpful.

Service users' views of practitioners

We wanted to establish what service users felt about the quality of practice they received from specialist palliative care social workers. We paid particular attention to exploring any negative views service users might have. We wanted to identify and avoid any tendency towards what has been called the 'grateful patient syndrome', whereby people at a difficult time in their life might be excessively positive about any help they receive, however limited. We also wanted to minimise the possibility of social workers who accessed service users to the project 'cherry picking' those who might have particularly positive views. For this reason, we included check questions in our interview/group discussion schedule to provide several opportunities to elicit negative views.

In the event, however, although we encouraged people to tell us about any negative views they might have about specialist palliative care social work, most participants found this question very hard to answer, generally because they felt their experiences had been so overwhelmingly positive. There was no evidence that this resulted from the process by which service users were included in the project. Although they struggled hard, only a few participants could think of any negative experiences. For example:

I was very angry with the social worker a lot of the time. I just felt I was being deserted, but it wasn't her fault. But you don't realise that until afterwards. You just need that contact even every couple of days... I just needed someone to let me know that something was happening.

(white UK bereaved woman, age group 46–55 years)

Because I couldn't get any help, anyone to mediate between me and the nursing home, I ended up taking charge of all her drugs and all her money and trying to sort everything out... At that time, my dealings with [the specialist palliative care social worker] *tended to tail off because it was making me more upset than it was helping.*

(no details available about the participant)

One woman was upset that a social worker had spoken to her in a corridor where they might have been overheard, and two people thought the social worker had not delved deep enough into their backgrounds and the issues facing them and their families. One of these had been referred by the social worker to a counsellor. But he did not find the counsellor very helpful and commented that he would much rather have talked to the social worker about his family.

One issue that did emerge in a very few instances was that service users highly valued the work of a particular social worker, but either knew others who had not done so, or it emerged in an interview that another service user was not so happy with the work of the same social worker. However, this was not a common theme.

Seeking feedback from service users

As part of our research, we wanted to find out whether service users had ever been asked what they thought of the service they received from the specialist palliative care social worker. An overwhelming majority of those we interviewed told us that they had never been asked to give any formal feedback or evaluation of the social work support they had received — or indeed of any other aspect of the hospice or specialist palliative care services they were receiving.

It was clear throughout the research that service users were asked informally and regularly by the social workers working with them whether they felt they were receiving appropriate support. This was part of the process of their relationship with the social worker and service users frequently commented on how, in their dealings with the specialist palliative care social worker, they felt they were able to determine the agenda.

However, in sharp contrast, more generally they had not been given any formal opportunity to give their views or evaluate the input of the specialist palliative care social worker in a way that could be fed back either to the wider multi-disciplinary team or to the management of hospice and specialist palliative care services within which the social workers were based. There are issues for palliative care management here.

Many services users who participated commented that the research was the first time they had ever been asked to give their views about the social worker and added that this was one reason they had agreed to take part. They valued the work of the social worker so highly they wanted to tell someone about it and they saw the interview as a vehicle for expressing their feelings. A few of those who were interviewed phoned up the social worker afterwards to insist on relating what they had said. Again, the participants of the steering group in the Midlands, who had previously been interviewed as members of a patient group, emphasised that they were keen to be interviewed again as they wanted to make sure we fully appreciated the excellent work done by the social worker at their hospice.

We asked people if they would have liked to have more formal opportunities for input, but most did not have strong views on this. Some appeared to link evaluation with complaining and commented that they would then have said something if they had been unhappy with the service they had received. One patient was concerned that giving formal feedback could be burdensome for those who are ill.

A sizeable minority said this was not an issue that they felt strongly about. However, it is one that has very important ramifications for the choices people have in receiving a social work service, a point to which we will return.

The organisation of palliative care social work

The lack of inquiry into what people thought about or wanted from specialist palliative care social work seemed to be linked to inconsistencies in its organisation and provision. Although we began our research with an interest in what service users wanted from specialist palliative care practice, we came to realise through the study that how this practice was experienced was inseparable from how it was organised and managed. While practice itself was essentially valued as positive, problems with its organisation and management began to emerge.

Our research revealed a lack of consistency throughout hospice and specialist palliative care services as to if, or when, service users and their families would get referred to, or see, the specialist palliative care social worker. Palliative care tends to be perceived as a valued service and there is evidence that access to it is unequal, notably in relation to ethnicity. However, even when people did reach the hospice or specialist palliative care unit, they could not be sure they would see a specialist social worker.

Many people said that it would have been helpful if they could have met the specialist palliative care social worker much earlier on in their journey through illness and all the problems and issues it can raise. Some felt it would have been helpful to meet such a social worker exactly at the time of diagnosis. One bereaved woman said:

> *I just wish that maybe that there's been someone like* [the specialist palliative care social worker] *around right from the word go... maybe through fault of our own, not knowing or not asking.*

(white UK bereaved woman, age group 26–35 years)

One woman expressed real regret on behalf of her husband, who had died some months earlier of a very virulent cancer. He was only referred to the hospice a few days before death. She had found the social worker so helpful to herself and her young children that she bitterly regretted that her husband had missed out on that help. By the time he arrived at the hospice, he was too ill to have more than the briefest of conversations with the social worker. Yet, she felt strongly that months before he needed someone to talk to outside the family who could perhaps have helped him face what he was going through.

Specialist palliative care social work support is not being offered, it seems, to patients and their families in a systematic, consistent way before the death of a patient. There was evidence of inconsistency even within the same unit. Sometimes, one service user told us that the social worker had been very proactive in offering support, whilst another user of the same hospice or palliative care team gave an opposing story of how they had needed to be very active in seeking out support (although it was clear that only a small minority of service users had themselves requested to see a social worker). Some social workers tried to meet all new patients — this was particularly common in day care settings.

Several people did slip through the net. One young bereaved woman told us how, despite frequent visits to the hospice while her sister was dying, she did not meet a social worker:

> *Whilst she was actually ill, I don't remember being introduced to them... I think it would have been easier if we had met them properly before she died.*

Referrals to the social worker frequently came through other professionals, but there was some evidence that those professionals were not always helpful and could act negatively as gatekeepers. One service user told us:

> *They actually said to me, 'Well, we've got a social worker here, but I don't actually think you'll like her and get on with her very well.' But having had contact with her I found her extremely good.*

This patient had not been put off meeting the social worker but wondered if other patients had, after having been told the same thing. It was clear that many of the people we spoke to had been desperate for support before they met the specialist palliative care social worker. As one service user said:

> *I just remember coming out of a black hole and that's how I described it seeing her face, and that was the first contact. And I don't know why, you know, I just don't know why, I just felt I had to talk to this person.*

Given the inconsistency in the way people are referred to the specialist palliative care social worker, one wonders how many others there are who do not get the support they need.

Implications for the future

The very positive views about specialist palliative care social work offered by service users in this study must be contrasted with the frequently negative views that have emerged about social work — specifically, child protection social work and social work with children and families. Most service users who participated in the project said that before their contact with the specialist palliative care social worker, they held negative views of social work and social workers generally. For a few, this was based on direct personal experience, but many admitted that they knew very little about what social workers really did and relied on the media for information:

> *I was a bit wary of them, can I put it that way? I think we are very influenced by what we read in the press... I thought they might be a bit intrusive into my life.*

> (white UK female patient, age group 56–65 years)

> *I thought social work was for the down-and-outs — people that, you know, lived on the streets and things like that.*

> (female patient talking in discussion group)

Such views may mean that some service users would be unlikely to request the specialist palliative care social work service that others later found so helpful.

Paradoxically, the wider professional recognition granted to specialist palliative care social work may be undermined by its strengths. One of the characteristics we noticed was the lack of professional trappings that accompanied the social work role, reflected in, for example, its flexibility, the lack of the role's strict definition, and the lack of a perceived hierarchy or formalised processes of referral and assessment. Service users welcomed these qualities and perceived them as strengths. However, until this study, unfortunately, little effort had been made to establish what service users think. As one woman service user said:

> *I think it would be nice if they did ask people, just so that people who came along afterwards benefit from that — you know, from other people's experiences... Tiny things can help a lot because it is so hard.*

But far from being universally available in palliative care, there are still some hospices and palliative care teams that do not have a dedicated social worker. New National Institute for Clinical Excellence (NICE) guidelines do not explicitly include social workers as core members of the palliative care team. The core team is identified as medical consultants, nurse specialists and administrators (NICE, 2004). Recently, a voluntary hospice disbanded its entire social work team.

Yet the Involve! study showed clearly that most service users felt that the support of the specialist palliative care social worker was essential for them and their families throughout their difficult journey through illness and bereavement. The specialist palliative care social worker was seen as offering a holistic service that was not offered by other professionals who worked with them. Others have echoed these findings of a distinctive role for social work within multidisciplinary teams (Herod and Lymbery, 2002). Research has also shown that the gaps service users have identified in both oncology and generalist palliative care services relate to social and psychological support (McIllmurray *et al*, 2001; Hill *et al*, 2003).

As yet, little notice seems to have been taken of what service users of specialist palliative care social work have to say and minimal efforts been made to gain their views. Until this happens, so that these can be included in service planning and development, and until service users are themselves more fully involved, we can only expect future patients and families to lose their opportunities to gain greatly valued support from specialist palliative care social work.

References

Balloch S, Beresford P, Evans C, Harding T, Heidensohn M, Turner M (1998) Advocacy, empowerment and the development of user-led outcomes. In: Craig YC (ed) *Advocacy, Counselling and Mediation in Casework*. Jessica Kingsley, London

Beresford P, Croft S, Evans C, Harding T (1997) Quality in personal social services: the developing role of user involvement in the UK. In: Evers A, Haverinen R, Leichsenring K, Wistow G (eds) *Developing Quality in Personal Social Services: Concepts, Cases and Comments*. European Centre Vienna. Ashgate, Aldershot

Beresford P, Broughton F, Croft S, Fouquet S, Oliviere D, Rhodes P (2000) *Palliative Care: Developing User Involvement, Improving Quality*. Centre for Citizen Participation, Brunel University

Harding T, Beresford P (eds) (1996) *The Standards We Expect: What Service Users and Carers Want from Social Services Workers*. National Institute for Social Work, London

Herod J, Lymbery M (2002) The social work role in multi-disciplinary teams. *Practice* **14**(4): 17–27

Hill KM, Amir Z, Muers MF, Connolly CK, Round CE (2003) Do newly diagnosed lung cancer patients feel their concerns are being met? *Eur J Cancer Care* **12**(1): 35–45

McIllmurray MB, Thomas C, Francis B, Morris S, Soothill K, Al-Hamad A (2001) The psychosocial needs of cancer patients: findings from an observational study. *Eur J Cancer Care* **10**(4): 261–9

Schalock RL (1995) *Outcome-Based Evaluation*. Plenum Press, New York

Shaping Our Lives National User Network, Black User Group (West London), Ethnic Disabled Group Emerged (Manchester), Footprints and Waltham Forest Black Mental Health Service User Group (North London) and Service Users' Action Forum (Wakefield) (2003) *Shaping Our Lives — from Outset to Outcome: What People Think of the Social Care Services They Use*. Joseph Rowntree Foundation, York

Turner M (1997) *Shaping Our Lives: Interim Report* (October). Shaping Our Lives, National Institute for Social Work, London

Turner M (1998) *Shaping Our Lives: Project Report* (October). Shaping Our Lives, National Institute for Social Work, London

Chapter 3

Culture and ethnicity — its relevance for social work practice in palliative care

Jane Thomson

Aya is frail and very near to death. She lies gently propped up by pillows with her face turned towards Mecca, surrounded by her sons and daughters. They softly pray with and for her; and Aya, now too weak to say the words herself, lifts her index finger as a sign of her presence. Shortly afterwards, she becomes unconscious. At the point of death, her family places a drop of water in her mouth, demonstrating their belief that death is not the end but signifies her entry into the world of the divine. 'That was as it should be — she will continue,' her eldest son later tells the hospice nurse.

This vignette gives a glimpse into death for devout Muslims, and some of the beliefs and traditions that accompany it (see Gatrad, 2002). It illustrates the significance of culture for the way we live and die, and how it lies at the heart of our beliefs, values and traditions. This chapter aims to define culture and ethnicity, their relevance for the total care model of palliative care in general, and for the social workers employed in this area in particular.

Culture and ethnicity

What is the relevance of culture and ethnicity for thought and practice in social work in twenty-first century Britain? What is certain is that issues of culture and ethnicity are not new. As the Commission for Racial Equality (CRW) points out (www.cre.gov.uk/ethdiv/ethdiv.html):

Britain has always been a mixed society — a nation peopled by migrants — from Bronze Age and Neolithic migrants who travelled to north-west Europe five thousand years ago, to the refugees from

eastern Europe and Africa arriving today. Most people in Britain are
either immigrants or the descendants of immigrants.

(Commission for Racial Equality)

The 2001 census gave information on the ethnic make-up of England and Wales. It found that 87% of the population of England and 96% of those living in Wales gave their ethnic origin as white British, and that London has the highest proportion of people from minority ethnic groups, apart from those of Pakistani origin who form 2.9% of the population of Yorkshire and the same proportion in the West Midlands. Of the other ethnic groups, 2% are Indian, 0.5% Bangladeshi and 1.1% black Caribbean; white Irish make up 1.2% of the total population.

The relevance of these figures is more evident when related to geographical area — for example, the Bangladeshi population in England and Wales is 0.5%, but clustered together in the London borough of Tower Hamlets, where they form 33.4% of the resident population. In Leicester, by contrast, 25.7% of the entire city's population is Indian.

Significantly, the census figures do not include the many other ethnic groups that make up England's (and, in particular, London's) diversity: Jews, Turks, Poles and those from south-east Asia to mention but a few.

Faith is another powerful determinant of culture and ethnicity, with 1.5 million Muslims forming the second largest religious group in England and Wales, while Hindus and Sikhs make-up the majority of the remaining ethnic-minority communities.

These minority communities are young populations with an above-average birthrate and therefore likely to grow in numbers in the years ahead. Culture and ethnicity, therefore, need to be firmly and increasingly on the country's agenda for the future.

So what are culture and ethnicity? What are the common features and how do they differ? First, culture. Helman (1994) defines it as:

> *a set of guidelines (both explicit and implicit) which individuals*
> *inherit as members of a particular society, and which tells them*
> *how to view the world, how to experience it emotionally, and how*
> *to behave in it in relation to other people, to supernatural forces or*
> *gods and to a natural environment. It also provides them with a way*
> *of transmitting these guidelines to the next generation — by the use*
> *of symbols, language, art and ritual.*

Culture gives a sense of identity through a shared language or group of languages, history and, above all, a set of shared beliefs, values and traditions. Culture, then, is not a singular concept, but a multi-faceted one: it provides different 'explanatory models' (Kleinmann, 1986) of how the world is, and how best to live, work, play and conduct relationships within it. Culture is what brings diversity to the world and makes its people such a rich tapestry. It generates strong loyalties and, where it is not understood and respected, can be the catalyst for tension and strife. One thing is certain: in the highly populated and mobile world of the twenty-first century, it will remain a central issue to be understood more deeply if greater equality and peace are to exist for all people.

How is culture separate from ethnicity? The latter has been defined as the means of describing a group of people who share characteristics that give them distinctiveness and a difference from others (Price and Cortis, 2000). Another definition (Field, Hockey and Small, 1997) states that 'ethnicity is generally agreed to refer to collective awareness of shared origins or descent and is a rational concept referring to a sense of identity as a member of a group and to difference from others'. This definition highlights the sense of belonging and group identity that gives ethnicity a more permanent core than the definitions of culture, which highlight behaviour and attitudes. But both definitions share a sense of individuality and suggest a psychological connection. Race, on the other hand, is characterised by genetic ancestry and evidenced in physical appearance. It is, however, a contested concept and one that has been replaced by ethnicity (Solomos, 2003; Solomos and Back, 1996). Indeed, this allows social workers to consider individual belief systems and group identities rather than work with the rigid and potentially oppressive stereotypes of race.

The fact that culture can evolve to meet the changing social environment is shown in our own society by the secularisation of death during the past few generations. In the past, the process of dying and death was deeply influenced by religion (mainly Christianity). Today, with a steep decline in those who actively hold a Christian or any other faith belief, death tends to be seen as the end of a person's life, rather than the beginning of a new one.

Another example of social evolution in the UK during the past century is the move from being a predominantly rural society, with a largely static population, to one that is urban-based with a highly mobile population, with the accompanying breakdown in the sense of community, lifestyle and traditions.

Equally, it is the mobility of the world's peoples that acts as a catalyst for the preservation of different cultures by different ethnic groups; it is fired by the same human need to belong to a group of like-minded people that brings those with a shared background to live together when they find themselves in societies that vary from their own. Many large cities now have geographical areas where people from different ethnic groups are based, and where their cultural traditions are upheld.

It is the ease of access to fast international travel for an ever-growing proportion of the world's population that has further enabled the exposure of more people to a range of different cultures and an appreciation of their richness and diversity. As a result, individuals' belief systems and lifestyles may change or whole communities may adapt to their evolving circumstances and experiences. Adversely, where an existing culture is threatened and dominated by that of an invading people who hold different beliefs and traditions, which may be imposed against the wishes of the indigenous population, the latter may flounder and wither. A powerful example is the Bushmen of the Kalahari whose homelands were reduced and laws imposed that seriously impeded their ability to live in their traditional way. Similarly, the Maoris of New Zealand, the Australian Aborigines and the Inuit peoples of Canada's coastal lands have had their lifestyles seriously threatened and eroded, and have struggled to maintain the sense of ethnic individuality and culture that accompanies it.

What is the relevance of culture and ethnicity to palliative care?

Multicultural societies, then, are not new. But the challenge for the twenty-first century is to find a way both to respect cultural diversity and to celebrate it, and to create equality of opportunity and participation for everybody living in the host nation.

In 1927, Peabody wrote:

What is spoken of as a 'clinical' picture s not just a photograph
of a man sick in bed: it is an impressionistic picture of the patient
surrounded by his home, his work, his relations, his friends, his joys,
sorrows, hopes and fears.

This was also the vision of Dame Cecily Saunders, the founder of the modern hospice movement and herself the embodiment of the multi-professional approach through her various educations as a nurse, social worker and doctor. It was through her work and that of her team that the notion of 'total pain' and the response of 'total care' was developed. This recognition of the need to respond to the whole person — their physical, emotional, intellectual, social and spiritual needs — through the care of a multi-professional team is now well-established. So if holistic care is to be fulfilled, the differing needs, wishes and aspirations of patients and their loved ones must be recognised and respected, and care provided in a sensitive way that meets them. This must also include 'culturally competent care'. As David Oliviere writes:

in an era when most societies in Europe are multicultural, if the
concepts of cultural pain and cultural care are not made explicit,
their importance in good patient care may be ignored.

Thus, awareness of peoples' differing ways of life, beliefs and traditions is imperative if palliative care is to be offered in a sensitive and appropriate way, and to be of a high standard. This is especially true now, at the beginning of the globalised twenty-first century, when multicultural societies are rapidly becoming the norm.

The importance of culture and ethnicity for social work practice

The importance of culture and ethnicity rests on the values that guide all good social work practice.

Cultural competence and safety

If a patient is to be understood as fully as possible, it is necessary to know and appreciate his or her culture and ethnic mores. But how is this to be achieved and integrated into practice? The concepts of 'cultural competence' (Leininger, 1996) and 'cultural safety' (Ramsden, 1993) are helpful in this respect. They recognise the need for understanding and acceptance of beliefs, values and behaviours of people from different ethnic groups, but also go beyond practical skills to include attitudinal change. As Firth explains, '[these concepts] insist on empowering the ethnic minorities themselves to be involved in the development of culturally safe practice in partnership with the majority community' (Coup, 1996). Thus, cultural safety aims to provide care that will 'recognise, respect and nurture the unique cultural identity... and safely meet their needs, expectations and rights' (Polaschek, 1998, cited in Oliviere, 1999). Cultural safety needs to be firmly grounded in the practice of every social worker if patients, their families and others close to them are to feel comfortable and secure in all aspects of their care.

During training, social work students are required to examine and become aware of their own values, beliefs and, importantly, prejudices. Only by doing so can they open themselves to learn about and accept the beliefs and values of other cultures in a non-judgemental way. This is fundamental for cultural competence. It is a process that should be continued throughout practice life through structured supervision, self-monitoring and feedback from colleagues and, hopefully, users of the service. Gunaratnam *et al* (1998) refer to this process as 'emotional labour'. Relevant questions might be, 'Am I being racist?' or 'Am I making appropriate cultural assumptions about needs and experiences?' Abram, Slosar and Walls (2005) develop these concepts further in a challenging way, using the term 'reverse mission' to emphasise the importance of learning from and listening to others in order to transform practice.

Also helpful in gaining this unbiased understanding is 'referential grounding': which involves:

> *identifying similar instances from one's own experience and*
> *knowledge and transferring the insight back to practice. It can*
> *involve real or imaginative comparisons with similar-case white*
> *individuals or families to enable empathetic understanding. This*

> *helps to identify ethnic-minority people, not as 'others', but with common needs and experiences.*

> Gunaratnam *et al* (1998)

The added understanding and insight gained by making comparisons in this way is an important basis for interpersonal communication. It enables one individual to see another, irrespective of race, culture and ethnicity, as a human being with common hopes, fears and aspirations for themselves and those close to them.

The danger of making assumptions

If palliative care is to be available to all people and experienced at an equally high standard, learning about different cultures, beliefs, values and traditions is essential. It can help us understand our patients' lives and act appropriately: it is what stops a white Christian social worker from feeling rejected when an orthodox-Jewish man does not shake hands with her; it is what helps us understand why a dying Asian woman who seems to need some peace is surrounded hour after hour by relatives and friends who come to pay their respects; it is what makes a social worker aware of the rights of the family rather than the individual, which prevails in many ethnic-minority groups.

But such knowledge also carries the danger of assuming that all members of the same ethnic group will choose to behave in the same way, and that their needs and wishes will be the same. Most people, whatever their ethnic group, have a tendency to generalise in order to make sense of their own experiences. This can easily lead to rigidity of thought and stigmatisation. In our highly mobile world, people of the same race frequently have very different life experiences that influence and mold their own cultural practises and outlook. In a phenomenological study by Diver, Molassiotis and Weeks (2003), the four ethnic minority patients attending day care expressed basic human needs rather than particular cultural ones, reflecting the need for sensitivity in responding to individuals and not working from received assumptions of cultural need.

For example, imagine that a middle-aged Indian woman is admitted to a hospice inpatient unit. She is frequently visited by her husband, children and other relatives and friends, many of whom are dressed in saris. The nurses assume she is Hindu and offer her a vegetarian diet. In reality, she has lived and worked in England all her life, is a devout Christian and is not vegetarian at all. Whilst her family are of great importance to her, she does not share the belief of many traditional Asian families that it is their sacred duty to care for a sick family member and that not to do so will result in 'loss of face' and stigmatisation for the family.

Equally misleading is the assumption that all service users are knowledgeable about their own needs, and can articulate them. For some, in particular those from ethnic-minority groups, there is a lack of understanding about the way health care is offered in Britain. The possibility of dialogue and debate with the doctor who is treating them is alien and frightening. For others, especially Asian women, the notion that their wishes could override those of their family, and in particular their husband, is equally difficult to grasp.

So culture is subtle, variable within the same group, and likely to evolve with different experiences and over time. Good social work practise finds the individuality of each person and the culture they inhabit. As Gunaratnam (1998) points out, it is necessary to go beyond the external difference and to relate to others as human beings. Her concepts of 'referential grounding' and 'emotional work' are helpful in this respect.

Working with difference is about discovering our common humanity, whilst respecting and celebrating its diversity. It is about first being comfortable with ourselves and being open to the constant challenges to our own beliefs and value-systems. It is also about reassessing and confirming them so that we are more confident in responding to the different needs of others (Dominelli, 2002). This is the challenge of working with people from cultures different from our own who are terminally ill and dying. Only this way can service providers be constantly aware of, and sensitive to, the needs of those who use their service.

Equality of access

Equality of access is the belief that everyone who needs a service should receive it, irrespective of culture, ethnicity or race. For this belief to be translated into practice, social work planners and practitioners require an accurate and up-to-date knowledge of the ethnic make-up of the community they serve, and of their differing needs and wishes without assuming homogeneity. When *Opening Doors* (1995) was researched and written, there was clear evidence that black and other ethnic-minority people were not receiving palliative care in proportion to their numbers. The findings of the 2001 population census showed that this situation was largely unchanged. As Firth (2001) writes in *Wider Horizons*:

> *The ethnic-minority population in 2001 is estimated to be around 10%, yet the figures provided by the Hospice Information Service for use of hospices and palliative care services in 1999–2000 show that 3% of recorded adult patients and 18% of children are from black and ethnic-minority communities.*

Although the absolute accuracy of this data remains unconfirmed (since it depends on individual palliative care services having completed their statistical returns accurately), it is indicative of the work that remains to be done if equality of access to palliative care services is to become a reality. It also reflects the situation in the USA where only 8% of those benefitting from hospice care services are from African-American communities (Winston *et al*, 2004).

Hill and Penso (1995) identified the reasons for poor service provision to ethnic-minority groups as:

- low referral rates
- lack of knowledge and information about services
- lower incidence of cancer in black ethnic groups
- the preference of many black and Asian families to care for the dying family members at home rather than using inpatient hospital or hospice services.

In 2005, this is still the case. Despite some marginal attempts, the provision of culturally sensitive care for ethnic-minority patients remains a concern for many service providers. Gradually, there is a growing awareness of this and a recognition of the need to improve culturally sensitive service delivery if it is to be accessible to everyone who needs it (Gatrad *et al*, 2003; Gatrad, 2002; Nyatanga, 2002). One effective way of hastening the process is by building relationships of openness and trust between service providers and the different ethnic communities through their organisations and community leaders. Such relationships should be ones of equality in which both parties work together to find ways to provide sensitive palliation that is appropriate for the differing needs of each community. An example is to find a way for black African and Caribbean people to mourn the death of a family member with their customary chanting and wailing at the hospice. Often, this 'style' of mourning is unintentionally distressing to patients and families from other ethnic backgrounds, unless explanations are offered and a safe place is found for the grief to be expressed in this way.

Anti-discriminatory practice

Anti-discriminatory practice is closely linked to equality of access and a consistent standard of service for all people. By definition, its aim is to ensure that no individual is barred from receiving the care they need because of their race, ethnicity, faith, gender, sex, age or any other reason. It requires a knowledge of relevant law, in particular the Race Relations (Amendment) Act (2000) and the Equal Opportunities Act (1991; amended 2000) coupled with a determination to address disadvantage and oppression where it exists. Central to this is 'advocacy': an essential skill for social workers if their clients are to be treated fairly and receive the service and support they need. Advocacy requires an empathetic understanding of those being represented, and an ever-present awareness of the accuracy (or not) of clients' perceived needs. Good communication is vital, which may require the help of interpreters (see 'Good communication' section). Owens and Randhawa (2004) consider anti-oppressive practice crucial to culturally competent and ethnically sensitive palliative care.

Individuality

Respect for individuality — that is, the right of each human being to live and die in the way they choose — is a fundamental principle of good social work practice in the UK. But whilst this is entirely appropriate for European communities, it may be less so for Asian and other ethnic-minority groups, in which the rights of the patient are strongly influenced by those of their family and even their community.

By contrast, the values of European cultures are heavily influenced by the autonomy of the individual. Awareness of these differences is important if care is to be sensitively provided. For example, an elderly Asian woman should be invited to choose a family member to be present during consultations with any member of the palliative-care team, including the social worker, and understanding should be shown if she subsequently defers to her husband.

There is a strong need in social work practice to treat each person according to his or her requirements and experiences, which runs contrary to the popular maxim, 'all people should be treated the same'. Each of us, irrespective of culture and ethnic background, has a right to access the help we require; in that, we are equal. What differs is the *manner* in which assistance is provided, for which the maxim 'equal but different' might be more helpful.

Acceptance

Acceptance and a non-judgemental attitude about the way a person chooses to live and to die are other basic requirements if care is to be offered in a culturally sensitive way. When these are combined with a real desire and enthusiasm for understanding the reasons for the choices made, the potential for a deeper and more productive relationship between the individual and the social worker is improved. For example, a patient may decide not to have treatment that has the potential to extend life. Such a choice belongs to the patient, and providing it is based on an accurate understanding of the possible outcomes, it should be accepted and respected by caregivers.

Honesty

Honesty is an integral part of respect and essential if social workers' relationships with patients and those close to them are to be ones of openness and trust. Establishing trust is crucial for successful palliative care. It is only when a patient or family really trust the professionals working with them that they can openly and honestly express their deeper wishes and feelings, whether they are fears or hopes. Honesty also includes being clear about what the service can and cannot offer its users.

Not lying is crucial. Patients have a right to know about their disease, its treatment, its progression and its probable outcome. But they do not have a duty to know if they choose not to. Providing patients with the information they seek in a way and at a pace that they can understand is a skill that all members of the palliative care team must develop. Social workers have an important role as advocates for patients in ensuring that cultural sensitivities are known and respected by the team as a whole.

Good communication

Good communication is central to successful palliative care and for the social worker it lies at the very heart of their work. It is about attentive listening, without which a patient's hopes, fears and wishes may not be clearly expressed or received. If this happens, the probability of the ensuing care being offered in the 'right' way — that is, the way that the patient and their family choose — is greatly reduced.

Effective communication can be complex and delicate, even when the patient and the team caring for them share the same language; when they do not, it is a potential minefield. It requires the intended meaning of a patient's or their family's words to be checked constantly to ensure that they have been correctly understood. Patients often speak of 'going home' or 'being ready to leave', rather than talk directly of their death. Such conversations are often difficult for native speakers of English; how much harder they must be for those who speak English as a second or even third language. Often, family members act as interpreters, but this carries the risk that they may become distressed when emotionally difficult issues arise or prohibit the patient from mentioning concerns for fear of upsetting their relatives.

The use of a professional interpreter is one solution, but this also has its hazards. Many interpreters are trained to provide a word-for-word translation and may not understand the health issues or medical settings relevant to the patient's situation. Equally, they may become distressed by the emotional content of many of the conversations that take place between the patient and the palliative care team members. Interpreters need to be trained and carefully prepared for such sensitive work, and to develop a specialism in it.

There are a growing number of schemes that use either bilingual health advocates to represent patients' interests or bilingual health or social workers who work with specific ethnic groups to bridge the gap between them and the services they require. Although such services remain geographically patchy, Silvera and Kapasi (2000) have shown that health advocacy is a 'thriving activity' in London, where the majority of ethnic groups have such a service. They counted 163 such organisations and the number continues to grow. These are heartening data but should not dampen the need for ethnic groups themselves to be more actively involved in the planning and delivery of services.

A further important aspect of effective communication is the provision of relevant information in a format that is readily accessible for those who need it. The language used should be easily understood by the recipient and not full of medical jargon. Written material needs to be in a range of languages and presented in a way that takes account of varying levels of understanding, especially about the structures of the NHS and social services, and the intricacies of relevant financial benefits and grants. New arrivals to the UK may, for example, have little understanding of the roles of GPs and hospital medical consultants, or the relationship between them. This relationship needs to be explained if patients are to have confidence in the teams of professionals with whom advanced progressive disease brings them into contact.

Whilst written information plays its part, the importance of verbal communication cannot be overemphasised. A significant number of members of ethnic groups, especially those of the older generation, do not read and rely on verbal communication for explanations of available services and their own disease and treatment. To offer them only written material is not only pointless, but can also cause embarrassment and to lead to barriers developing in future contact. Help from cultural or religious centres for ethnic-minority groups is one way forward. Another is the use of advocates, link workers and professionally trained and well-supported volunteers, and there is a growing number of initiatives to develop this further.

Developing effective communication remains a challenge for social workers, but one which, when met with care, imagination and sensitivity, can be particularly rewarding.

Conclusion

Cultural and ethnic diversity brings richness to our society. To make palliative care available to every individual, in a way with which they are comfortable, requires imagination, sensitivity and creativity. Social workers, like all service providers, must recognise and respect differences between individuals, but also look beyond it to their shared humanity. Listening to patients and their families, and continually appraising their own attitudes and behaviour, are the ways to achieve this. Above all, there must be a genuine desire to communicate openly and honestly with patients, their families and carers. In this way, the richness of diversity will be preserved and any tensions seep away. Achieving success in what is undeniably a complex and demanding environment is rewarding for everybody. It was summed up by a black mother with three young children who had recently arrived from Africa with advanced cancer. After meeting her white social worker several times, she said: 'She understands me and what I want for my family. We are working together to make sure it happens.'

References

Abram FY, Slosar JA, Walls R (2005) Reverse mission: a model for international social work education and transformative intranational practice. *Int Soc Work* **48**(2): 161–76

Coup A (1996) Cultural safety and culturally congruent care: a comparative analysis of Irhapeti Ramsden's and Madeleine Leininger's educational projects for practice. *Nurs Prax NZ* **11**(1): 4–11

Diver F, Molassiotis A, Weeks L (2003) The palliative care needs of ethnic minority patients attending a day-care centre: a qualitative study. *Int J Palliat Nurs* **9**(9): 389–96

Dominelli L (2003) *Anti-Oppressive Social Work Theory and Practice*. Palgrave, Basingstoke

Field D, Hockey J, Small N (1997) *Death, Gender and Ethnicity*. Routledge, London

Firth S (2001) *Wider Horizons — Care of the Dying in a Multicultural Society*. National Council for Hospice and Specialist Care Services, London

Gatrad AR (2002) Palliative care for Muslims and issues before death. *Int J Palliat Nurs* **8**(11): 526–31

Gatrad AR, Brown E, Notta H, Sheikh A (2003) Palliative care needs of minorities. *BMJ* **327**(7408): 176–7

Gunaratnam Y (1997) Culture is not enough: a critique of multi-culturalism in palliative care. In: Field D, Hockey J, Small N (eds) *Death, Gender and Ethnicity*. Routledge, London

Gunaratnam Y (1998) Re-thinking multicultural service provision. *Hospital Bulletin* Aug 1998

Gunaratnam Y, Lewis G (2001) Racialising emotional labour and emotionalising racialised labour: anger, fear and shame in social welfare. *J Soc Work Pract* **5**: 2

Helman C (1994) *Culture, Health and Illness*. Butterworth-Heinemann, Oxford

Hill D, Penso D (1995) *Opening Doors: Improving Access to Hospice and Specialist Palliative Care Services by Members of the Black and Ethnic Minority Communities*. National Council for Hospice and Specialist Palliative Care Services, Occasional Paper 7

Kleinmann A (1986) *Social Origins of Distress and Disease: Neurasthenia and Pain in Modern China*. Yale University Press, New Haven

Leininger M (1996) Response to Cooney article, 'a comparative analysis of transcultural nursing and cultural safety'. *Nurs Prax NZ* **11**(2): 13–15

Nyatanga B (2002) Culture, palliative care and multiculturalism. *Int J Palliat Nurs* **8**(5): 240–6

Office of Population Censuses and Surveys (OPCS) (2001) *Census 2001*. National Report for England and Wales

Oliviere D (1999) Culture and ethnicity. *Eur J Palliat Care* **6**: 2

Owens A, Randhawa G (2004) 'It's different from my culture: they're very different': providing community-based 'culturally competent' palliative care for South Asian people in the UK. *Health Soc Care Community* **12**(5): 414–21

Parkes CM, Laungani P, Young B (eds) (1997) *Death and Bereavement across Cultures*. Routledge, London

Peabody FW (1927) The care of the patient. *JAMA* **88**: 12

Polaschek NR (1998) Cultural safety: a new concept in nursing people of different ethnicities. *J Adv Nurs* **27**(3): 452–7

Price KM, Cortis JD (2000) The way forward for transcultural nursing. *Nurse Educ Today* **20**(3): 233–43

Ramsden I (1993) Cultural safety in nursing education in Aotearoa (New Zealand). *Nurs Praxis NZ* **8**(3): 4–10

Saunders C (ed) (1990) *Hospice and Palliative Care: an Interdisciplinary Approach*. Edward Arnold (Hodder and Stoughton), London

Silveri M, Kapasi R (2000) *Health Advocacy for Minority Ethnic Londoners: Putting Services on the Map?* Kings Fund/NHS Executive, London

Solomos J (2003) *Race and Racism in Britain*. Palgrave, Basingstoke

Solomos J, Back L (1996) *Racism and Society*. Macmillan, Basingstoke

Winston C, Leshner P, Kramer J, Allen G (2004) Overcoming barriers to access and utilization of hospice and palliative care services in African-American communities. *Omega: J Death Dying* **50**(2): 151–63

Chapter 4

Working together — a multidisciplinary concern

Judith Hodgson

Introduction

Multidisciplinary and interdisciplinary work are terms frequently used, if not overused, in social work practice. They are words that trip off the tongue so easily that occasionally their meaning might be misunderstood, misconstrued, or even misused. When we use them what do we really mean? Do we mean 'teamwork', 'co-working', or any number of other terms with a similar meaning? Furthermore, they may be construed as 'quantitative' statements and the place of 'quality' in their application needs some analysis. In social work, multidisciplinary work is being actively promoted and recognised as part of the required value base under which we practice. The General Social Care Council Code of Practice for Employees (GSCC, 2002: 6.5) states that

> *social care workers must work openly and co-operatively with colleagues and treat them with respect*

and 6.7 takes this further:

> *Social care workers are also required to recognise and respect the roles and expertise of workers from other agencies and work in partnership with them.*

It is also the case that, whilst interprofessional working is generally promoted and indeed forms part of the new curriculum for social work education, it is not something that has been well-researched. Inquiries tell us that not working collaboratively leads to failures (Laming, 2003), but research does not necessarily tell us that collaborative working is effective or in what ways it might be so. In this chapter, I will look closely at the terms 'multidisciplinary work' and 'interdisciplinary work' and discuss how they are applied in practice with particular reference to the hospice in which I work. I will look at aspects of hospice social work practice that give multidisciplinary and interdisciplinary working quality as well as quantity, but I will also suggest areas where quality might be wanting and improvements made.

In this chapter, I will use the terms 'patient', 'client' and 'service user' interchangeably. While this may raise a number of objections, it locates the discussion in the multiprofessional and multidisciplinary base of the hospice.

Exploring the terms

The term 'multidisciplinary working' fills me with foreboding. I have visions of patients, usually in hospital or hospice beds, surrounded by swarms of different members of the helping professionals and being overwhelmed by their benevolence. Of course, the patients have no voice in this nightmare scenario. They are bombarded with advice, guidance, reassurance, bad news, instructions and questions. Furthermore, these professionals do not talk to each other. Each is working on his or her own — but of course, with the 'best interests' of the clients or patients at heart, whatever that may mean.

A different vision may arise when considering 'interdisciplinary working'. In this picture, 'worthies' once again surround our patients, but this time they talk to each other and plan together. What is more important is that they are also talking to the patients; their views and opinions are being listened to, together with those of their carers and families. In both these scenes, 'multi' implies many and 'inter' implies a collaboration between people.

The above discussion highlights the need to properly define what we mean by such terms and phrases (Payne, 2000). In the present chapter, we need to discuss how these terms relate to social work in hospices and how they affect the patient. There are so many questions and doubts that arise from the use of these terms, yet the processes they describe are usually thought to be the best way of working. The implication is that this way of working is always of benefit to the client and central to the modernising agenda in health and social care (Health Act, 1999; Whittington, 2003a, b). This is also the case in palliative care social work in which teamwork is generally considered to be positive (Sheldon, 1997). However, we still need evidence to support multidisciplinary and interprofessional working (Weinstein, Whittington and Leiba, 2003).

I have already suggested that the term 'multi' is quantitative. Some patients with palliative care needs have a whole array of professional people working with them, but some may have only one or two and others may rely solely on their GP for care. For some patients, therefore, multidisciplinary working is not the chosen way forward and the benefits of simpler and less quantitative care should not be discounted. It is important here to ensure that further research into the qualitative aspects of interdisciplinary working is undertaken from the perspective of service users rather than professionals and policy planners (see Barton, 2003; Douek, 2003; and *Chapter 2*).

The terms 'multidisciplinary' or 'interdisciplinary' are often used synonymously. Whilst 'professional' suggests members of distinct groups working together, when 'multi-' or 'inter-' are linked with 'disciplinary' it may relate more to skills and knowledge bases (Payne, 2000). Yet whichever of these terms we use, the concern is with collaboration or cooperation within their roles rather than with seeking to cross boundaries (Payne, 2000: 9). 'Inter-' is more qualitative, meaning 'between, among, in the midst of, mutual, reciprocal, together'. This definition does not emphasise the numbers of professionals involved, but rather how they do what they do.

> *Interprofessional, interdisciplinary… imply that professional groups make adaptations in their role to take account of and interact with the roles of others.*

> (Payne, 2000: 9)

Some 'role blur' and permeability is bound to occur in this way of working. For social workers, as for other professionals, the central matter to be aware of is how one retains a strong sense of professional identity.

The terms used remain contested and, as Leathard (1993) points out, we roam a 'semantic quagmire' in explaining them. If we consider how multiprofessional and multidisciplinary teams work in practice, we will be in a better position to understand them from the palliative care perspective.

We must also ask who decides the membership of this group of practitioners. The NICE Guidance distinguishes between core members and other members, and social workers appear to be optional core members. This is unhelpful and encourages neither multidisciplinary nor interdisciplinary working, but perhaps also reflects — and encourages — a hierarchy of care. Social work has had a troubled history, which struggles against antipathy from Government and the general public (Lymbery, 2004). These external pressures are matched by internal insecurities. I remember my first lecture on a social work/social administration course in 1972 in which social work was labelled a 'semi-profession' because it did not have a body of knowledge comparable to those of the more traditional professions, such as law or medicine. Much has been written in the last thirty years, but I am not sure if social work as a profession has progressed far, and new initiatives such as Sure Start have not had full social work involvement. The identity of social work is possibly a healthier one in the voluntary sector where, and perhaps surprisingly, economic restrictions on practice are not as rigorous.

A hospice experience

I manage a multidisciplinary team of social workers, all of whom have different roles and responsibilities within the hospice, a chaplain and volunteers. The social workers in our team have had similar training, yet have a different range of skills and roles. We then fit into a larger multiprofessional team consisting of doctors, nurses, physiotherapists, complementary therapists and volunteers. In addition, we must not omit the vital support systems such as administrators and secretaries, catering staff and ancillary staff internal to the hospice.

We must then include those who are external to the hospice if the work is to be truly multidisciplinary or collaborative. Therefore, we have to include GPs, other hospital services especially nurse practitioners, social services, DSS, occupational therapists (if not internal), charities, Community Macmillan nurses, district nurses, dentists and chiropodists. This arrangement is already messy and we have not yet included the service user or carers, who are central to effective and ethical collaborative working (see *Figure 4.1*).

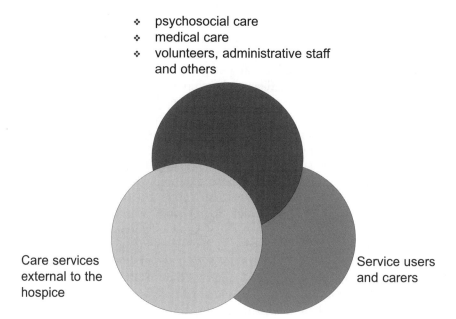

The hospice team:

❖ psychosocial care
❖ medical care
❖ volunteers, administrative staff and others

Care services external to the hospice

Service users and carers

Figure 4.1: Multiple involvement in hospice

Discharge planning meetings (DPM)

Sometimes, interdisciplinary working in the hospice is obvious, sometimes less so. An example of 'obvious' working is in the Discharge Planning Meeting

(DPM). These quite formal meetings are called when a discharge is particularly complicated, especially when there is involvement of young children, mental health issues, or difficulties in providing care at home. A member of the social work team will chair the meeting and advocate for the patient and family. This is not easy and it may be asked — how can fairness and objectivity be maintained when the chair is also acting on behalf of the person for whom the meeting has been called? Despite concerns, this dual role, which has evolved over many years, seems to work. In the absence of an independent chair, it is usually believed that the social worker is the best person available to assimilate all the facts of the case brought by the other professionals present and incorporate too the psychosocial issues.

> *'I think what is valuable is you just having a broader, all-encompassing view of the community and the people and what's out there. A much wider picture than some of the other disciplines.'*

(Herod and Lymbery, 2003: 4)

This meeting can involve a huge assortment of professionals, alongside the patient and family, all trying to find the best way forward. From within the hospice, there will be the named nurse, a physiotherapist, possibly someone from Day Therapies Unit, a social worker in the chair, and the patient with members of his or her family. (A doctor will most likely be invited but will rarely attend.) From outside, we will probably have invited the district nurse involved and representatives from adult social services. We have a captive audience of all those connected with the future care of the patient and a good 'chair' will allow everyone present to speak and then, together, draw up a list of recommendations — the 'best fit' of which will determine future care. An example of a list of recommendations would be as follows:

1. Patient to be discharged home on a specific date (or whenever services are in place).
2. District nursing services to visit daily.
3. Social services to provide a 'Getting up' and 'Going to bed' service.
4. Social services to arrange night sitters (Marie Curie) and to liaise with the family who will cover other nights.
5. Day sitters to be considered once or twice a week to give the carer a break.
6. Day care services (one day per week) to be offered, plus respite care and pain and symptom control care when needed after discharge.
7. Counselling support to be offered to the family and patient.

Thus, services are offered to the client and family or carers that best meet their needs at that time from a variety of professionals who work in a variety of agencies. They are aware of their own responsibilities and those of the others involved in the patients' care. All who attend the meeting have a time-limit to fulfil these responsibilities and furthermore each person receives a copy of the minutes. Everyone is aware of what everyone else is expected to do and regular and close communication is encouraged. If some recommendations cannot be fulfilled, further discussion is advised and the meeting will be reconvened.

In-patient multidisciplinary team meetings

Other examples of 'obvious' multidisciplinary working are the weekly multidisciplinary meetings (MDMs), where we look closely at the current patients on the Bedded Unit and the patients on Day Therapies Unit who are new, and those for whom there is particular concern.

The MDM involves another combination of professionals — nurses, doctors, a physiotherapist, the Day Therapies Coordinator (not surprisingly, Day Therapies patients are often regular in-patients and the presence of the coordinator ensures continuity of care and sharing of appropriate information), social workers, the chaplain, complementary therapists and a pharmacist. In this meeting, the issues of all the in-patients are discussed at length and plans made to tackle the issues.

However, we have recently had concerns that this way of working is not truly collaborative. All too often the weight of nursing and medical issues, alongside time-limitations, has meant that other contributions from other disciplines go unheard. Our initial response to these concerns is to have a chair for these weekly meetings, especially as the professional mix is growing: we have recently employed a lead complementary therapist and are seeking to appoint an occupational therapist, and it is vital that all areas of service user need are discussed.

We have mixed feelings about this course of action and will review the chair's role in a few months. In my opinion, it excessively formalises and makes business-like something that also needs to have elements of an open discussion. Perhaps as it settles down, a 'chair' structure will develop that embodies both open discussion and direction.

Plans and decisions are reworked as the patient's illness progresses in the three-times-daily nursing handover meetings. The significance of these meetings cannot be over-emphasised. They occur three times a day, seven days a week. In one week, therefore, there will be twenty-one meetings where accurate and up-to-date information about the patients and their carers will be shared. This is a huge opportunity to ensure continuity of multidisciplinary and interdisciplinary care, but all too often it is missed and only nurses are present.

Day-patient multidisciplinary meetings

The Day Therapies Unit cares for up to twenty-five patients each day. To discuss the needs of all these patients in depth, and in the time allotted in one meeting, would be impossible. The Day Therapies Unit therefore has its own interdisciplinary approach and a daily meeting takes place involving the Day Therapies Unit Coordinator, nurses, care assistants, a social worker, volunteers, an art therapist, a complementary therapist and very shortly an occupational therapist to discuss the patients expected that day and issues that might arise.

The population of day therapies is more stable and time is less of a concern. Some of the patients with neurological conditions have been attending for some time, and there are many opportunities as the weeks progress to discuss concerns that the patients or their families might have.

Sometimes, the work or communication with patients and their carers is not as fully or clearly documented as in DPMs and MDMs. Liaison with nurses and other professionals involved in a patient's care may not have the detailed luxury offered by these more formal meetings, but there should nevertheless be a trail of evidenced decisions (telephone calls, notes of conversations, etc) in the patient's notes/care plans. The importance of the more informal connections should not be forgotten. The 'best fit' will be less easily discernible, but it will be there, and may be clearer if shared notes are kept.

The best fit

I borrow the term 'the best fit' from Gerard Egan (2002). He devised a method of problem-solving, a working tool that is perhaps under-used in hospice social work. As social workers, we can get bogged down in psychological interventions or interventions that at the very least have psychological roots and we bypass interventions that have a more practical basis. Walter (1996) expressed a similar concern, which resulted in a shift in our thoughts on bereavement from a psychological emphasis to a sociological one.

Egan's (2002) method identifies three stages in reaching a solution to a particular problem:

1. Telling and exploring the story, identifying the issues that are causing concern and, finally, choosing a particular issue to work on. Where this is undertaken collaboratively, it prevents duplication and ensures that the service user's voice is paramount.
2. Focusing further on the chosen issue.

3. Exploring and identifying alternatives and solutions. This might involve a number of scenarios, some ideal and some unrealistic, and it is important to consider which are likely to be achievable. It is crucial at this stage that the service user directs this process.

An example in hospice social work might be when a dying person wants to address a previously unresolved issue with a family member. This issue might go back years, but for some reason has remained unresolved. The person may ask, 'Is it worth it?' Resolution may well bring peace of mind, but by taking this action it may add to the burden faced by those remaining after the service user's death. If the service user considers action to be worthwhile, social workers in particular may assist him or her through the process. This can bring structure to both collaborative working and decision-making for all involved, and in palliative care, when emotions are often close to the surface, this is surely a good thing.

However, there are also times when, despite all efforts to put together a full and appropriate package of care, things go wrong; or, at least, things do not go according to plan. A good example would be Client P, who suffers from multiple sclerosis (see below).

Case study 1: Client P

P has suffered from multiple sclerosis for some years and her condition is worsening physically and exacting a tremendous emotional toll as well. From a multiprofessional and multidisciplinary point of view, this case has the hallmarks of a good example. There are social workers, district nurses, GPs, consultant neurologists and urologists, hospice doctors, nurses, physiotherapists and alternative therapists involved through the hospice. A specialist in multiple sclerosis and a band of volunteers are also available. P's family, especially her husband, is also involved. We all communicate. We share information, and decisions are taken with full facts and P's full involvement.

Yet it is not ideal. There are emotional and psycho-spiritual issues that cannot be tackled because of our inability to master P's ever-changing physical symptoms. These issues include the death of a dearly loved son some years ago after years of illness; others include her relationship with her husband and the transition from a husband-and-wife relationship to a patient-and-carer one.

This case study indicates that even when many services are in place and working together, the result may not always be favourable. We have quantity, but not necessarily quality. To use a football analogy, the players are not working together as a team and they each have their own specific role to play, which can be achieved without relating to the other players. It is possible that in P's case, the 'multi' working has come about by accident, as the problems increased more and more specialists were brought in, but, unfortunately, effective communication has decreased. However, a second case study, of Mary, shows how interdisciplinary collaboration can be effective within the hospice.

Case study 2: Mary

Mary is in her late twenties. She is married with two children who are both under five years-old. A diagnosis of breast cancer with secondary spread has meant that curative treatment is no longer an option. She is admitted to a hospice for terminal care — a hospice that is proud of its multidisciplinary approach.

Early intervention from all disciplines (GP, district nurse, Community Macmillan Nurse, an Oncology Health Centre and social work or counselling support) mean that Mary and her family know the main people involved, and the consistency and continuity is welcome. Having been admitted to the hospice for pain and symptom control, she is already aware of the people treating and working with her. They have built up constructive working relationships with each other and her family. The latter will continue throughout the period of bereavement support.

Hospice care is supposed to offer palliative care at its best. However, palliative care does not end with the death and bereavement care is an integral part of palliative care. Bereavement care, furthermore, does not begin at the point of death; it should begin at the point of diagnosis of a life-limiting illness.

A vital component of the bereavement support offered to Mary's family will be that the bereavement services have known Mary. The person they hear about will be someone they knew. which will remove many barriers to communication. This fits into Walter's 'biography theory' (1999), which recognises that bereavement work is about telling the story of the person who has died, as well as sharing feelings.

Achieving quality

Case study 1 illustrates a quantitative multiprofessional approach to palliative care. I indicated that quality was lacking as a result of all these approaches; although they are very good in themselves, they are not coming together or communicating effectively. *Case study 2* shows how a quality service could be achieved. There are other ways of improving quality and standards of working collaboratively, some of which I will detail below.

Communication

Davy and Ellis (2000) point out that just because many people are involved does not mean that things will not be forgotten or that assumptions will not be made that someone else is taking on a particular responsibility or task. The watchword for effective multidisciplinary team working is 'communication'. It needs to be closely monitored; decisions should be reviewed regularly; and responsibility for action as a result of these decisions should be allocated clearly.

Effective communication leads to effective collaboration, the end result of which might be that the patient's quality of life, as well as that of the carers, will be improved. Unfortunately, communication between professionals does not necessarily guarantee clarity when communicating with service users. Jargon can confuse, create distance and emphasise an expert/patient relationship. Indeed, power relations are a much-ignored issue in multidisciplinary working in general. To be effective, we need to be clear, jargon-free, and take the time to explain the different roles that we have. To do this, of course, we need to be sure of our own roles in the first place.

Consistency

Davy and Ellis (2000) suggest that having many people involved in patient care can disrupt the relationships they have with other trusted professionals. Family life can also be disrupted by the many comings and goings of a range of helpers. In my experience, patients have gone home with the minimum of services because they did not want their homes turned into 'Piccadilly Circus', with the further obligation of having to be polite and make cups of tea for all people who come in and go out of their lives.

Furthermore, these professional helpers may vary from shift to shift and week to week and may not know the clients or each other. This lack of consistency of personnel is an issue that needs attention if we are to provide a quality service. If we are to achieve it, we need to communicate effective as a multidisciplinary team. In the hospice, it is possible to offer this limited and consistent approach to care.

Hierarchies

Disciplinary hierarchies can seriously disrupt the potential for effective multidisciplinary working. All professionals have a distinct identity and in some this may create a belief that their work is more important than that of a colleague. Sharing expertise and working together does not come easily. One's identity and knowledge-base may have been hard won, and what appears to be its 'dilution' is often an unpopular option.

At my own hospice, despite years of making my colleagues in other professions aware of psychosocial needs, and despite usually excellent and effective working relationships between all disciplines, there are times when I am convinced that old hierarchies remain. Of course, there is no point trying to look for them, especially not when the patient is wracked with pain or in acute discomfort. Nevertheless, the frustration is enormous when, once again, emotional and social needs are neglected.

Professional 'preciousness' can be seen in palliative care practice where representatives from one profession may put forward one point of view but not acknowledge that of other professionals. This is a limited and dangerous approach. At all times, we need to promote a truly interdisciplinary approach that is more productive and patient-centred.

Confidentiality

There are perceived risks to confidentiality where a number of different disciplines are involved in the same case and each of these disciplines might have a different interpretation of events. We need to ensure that the information we obtain is only that which will ensure the best possible care from our particular discipline.

But this is not easy, especially when there may only be one set of working notes. At the hospice where I work, much information is given to the psychosocial team that does not need to be shared. The other professionals acknowledge that there may be times when we obtain facts that they do not need to know, or which they just accept that the client does not wish anyone else to know. Equally, there will be areas of the patient's care that the psychosocial team do not need to know. Preserving confidentiality on a 'need to know' basis does not preclude multiprofessional working, but we need to be clear how, when and why we will share information and ensure that our clients are aware of these criteria.

Issues of time

With palliative care, we do not always have the luxury of time. Cicely Saunders (1990, 1999) tells us that time in palliative care situations is not merely to be understood as a 'quantity', but is rather a matter of 'depth' and 'quality'. If the patient has a poor prognosis, then the need is to make the best combination of decisions with them as quickly as possible and constantly to review these. If the social work team did not meet the patient and family until late in the course of the illness, a less then ideal social work service or bereavement service is likely to be offered. If a full and effective social work service is to be offered by hospice or palliative care social workers, there must be early referral to the service and this is only likely if there is an effective multidisciplinary and interdisciplinary system of working in place.

Issues of age

Some professionals believe that palliative care is only for older people who are facing the end of their lives (see *Chapter 1*). With younger patients, active treatment may continue until the point of death. This is understandable in a number of ways. The medical profession has a long history of wanting to make better, to cure (Parker, 2001). To acknowledge that this is no longer possible is not easy to communicate to the patient and the family. A switch of perception is required, involving a move away from maintaining life to ensuring that its end is as comfortable and dignified as possible, no matter what the age of the patient. This requires a great deal of courage from any professional, especially if the patient has a young family and under other circumstances a whole life ahead of them. However, this difficulty should not prevent the decision being made as it is vital, often, to developing an effective multidisciplinary response.

Issues of organisational difference

Working in a hospice, I believe that palliative care social work, at its best, can be found in our hospices. However, to be uncritical would be naïve and to see hospice care through 'rose-coloured spectacles'.

All hospices are different. They offer different services and have different emphases of care. Some have medical directors who can develop hospice services within the mainstream NHS services. Some have medical directors and boards of trustees who are happy that their service runs in a more independent way. Some hospices only have day units; some have extensive day and in-patient units. Some have teams of social workers; some only have one. Some employ counsellors. Some social work teams offer only bereavement care, some only in-patient care. Some teams offer only benefits advice and some offer a full range of services and complementary therapies with the support of teams of volunteers working alongside the medical and nursing professional staff. In my opinion, not enough offer full family and patient care from the point of diagnosis.

Hospices are funded mostly by voluntary contributions and although this brings the uncertainty of whether there is enough money coming in to continue to function 365 days per year, it also guarantees a level of independence from our public-sector financiers. The choice is therefore financial security or independence. Most hospices lie somewhere between these two extremes. The differences between organisations means that multidisciplinary and multiprofessional alliances and working will differ from hospice to hospice.

Geography

Information technology is increasingly important in health and social care (Rafferty and Waldman, 2003). Yet in multidisciplinary working these technologies cannot substitute for sharing an office or a building with different professionals. Walking down a corridor to discuss a client's progress face to face with a colleague is immediate, and we cannot be sure that e-mails or messages have been picked up.

Some years ago, the Community Macmillan Team were based at, and part-funded by, the hospice where I am employed. Members of the team were easily accessible — in their offices, the canteen, the car-park and generally around the hospice. Communication was not just easy — it could not be avoided! Joint visits, case discussions, early referrals and updates after a patient was discharged home were features of normal practice. Furthermore, there was little duplication as we had an awareness of each others' caseloads. The Community Macmillan Team moved out into the community and joint collaborative working became less easy to achieve. Meetings to discuss patients now need time, effort and synchronised diaries. However, we maintain good working relationships with all our Macmillan colleagues partly because of the joint working established in the early days when the 'geography' was in our favour.

Education

I have mentioned the 'preciousness' of individual professions earlier in this chapter. If this is to be reduced, early affirmation of collaborative working at the time of training might be helpful. Palliative care education (if not all education) and training for the caring professions must therefore be less precious also. Joint courses and projects and opportunities to learn and share ideas together at the time of training are vital if effective multidisciplinary and interdisciplinary working is to be achieved. This is encouraged in the new requirements for social work education (Department of Health, 2002; see also *Chapter 1*).

Conclusion

Cicely Saunders (1990) gave us the idea of 'total pain', which tells us that pain need not only be physical. A multidisciplinary approach gives this concept practical form by acknowledging that the patient and family are struggling with a number of different issues, all of which need to be looked into.

In an ideal world, hospice social work support would be available from the point of diagnosis alongside other services, and an effective working relationship built up between the helper, the patient and family that would continue after the death with bereavement support. Although palliative care is wider than cancer, the wish expressed in the NHS Cancer Plan (NHS, 2000) is poignant:

> *We want patients and their families to be confident that they will receive the information, support and specialist care they need from the time that cancer is first suspected through the subsequent stages of the disease. Good communication between health professionals and patients is essential.*

The *Guidance on Cancer Services: Improving Supportive and Palliative Care for Adults with Cancer* (NHS, 2004) recommends that comprehensive and holistic assessment of patients' needs should be an on-going process and that multidisciplinary team working is central to this:

> *Key Recommendation 3: Each multidisciplinary team or service should implement processes to ensure effective interprofessional communication within teams and between them and other service providers with whom the patient has contact. Mechanisms should be developed to promote continuity of care, which might include the nomination of a person to take on the role of 'key worker' for individual patients.*

There is no way that we can or should avoid working together. Good palliative care is a total care response to total pain and involves professions dealing with all aspects of human life. There is a delightful jigsaw puzzle in *Feeling Better* (Dix and Glickman, 1997), a discussion paper from the National Council for Hospice and Specialist Palliative Care Services. In the puzzle, the central piece, the patient, is surrounded by four interlinked 'care' pieces: spiritual, practical, psychosocial and physical. If one is removed, the overall picture is incomplete. Effective multidisciplinary and interdisciplinary care ensure that this puzzle remains complete, and it is this jigsaw that we need to promote in social work with people receiving palliative care and their families.

References

Barton C (2003) Allies and enemies: the service user as care coordinator. In: Weinstein J, Whittington C, Leiba T (eds) *Collaboration in Social Work Practice.* Jessica Kingsley, London

Davy J, Ellis S (2000) *Counselling Skills in Palliative Care.* Open University Press, Buckinghamshire

Department of Health (DoH) (2002) *Requirements for Social Work Training.* DoH, London

Dix O, Glickman M (1997) *Feeling Better: Psychosocial Care in Specialist Palliative Care: a Discussion Paper.* National Council for Hospice and Specialist Palliative Care Services, London

Douek S (2003) Collaboration or confusion? The carers' perspective. In: Weinstein J, Whittington C, Leiba T (eds) *Collaboration in Social Work Practice.* Jessica Kingsley, London

Egan G (2002) *The Skilled Helper: a Problem-Management and Opportunity-Development Approach to Helping.* 7th edn. Brookes/Cole, Pacific Grove, Ca

GSCC (2002) *Code of Practice for Employers and Employees.* GSCC, London

Laming H (2003) *The Victoria Climbié Inquiry Report.* Cmnd no. 5730. The Stationery Office, London

Leathard A (1994) *Going Interprofessional.* Routledge, London

Lymbery M (2004) Responding to crisis: the changing nature of welfare organisations. In: Lymbery M, Butler S (eds) *Social Work Ideals and Practice Realities.* Palgrave, Basingstoke

Herod J, Lymbery M (2003) The social work role in multidisciplinary teams. *Practice* **14**: 4

NHS (2000) *The NHS Cancer Plan: a Plan for Investment, a Plan for Reform.* NHS, London

NHS (2004) *Guidance on Cancer Services: Improving Supportive and Palliative Care for Adults with Cancer: the Manual.* National Institute for Clinical Excellence (NICE), London

Payne M (2000) *Teamwork in Multiprofessional Care.* Palgrave, Basingstoke

Parker J (2001) Interrogating person-centred dementia care in social work and social care practice. *J Soc Work* **1**(3): 329–45

Rafferty J, Waldman J (2003) *Building e-Learning Capacity for the Social Work Degree: a Scoping Study for the Department of Health e-Learning Steering Group.* DoH, London

Saunders C (1990) *Hospice and Palliative Care: an Interdisciplinary Approach.* Edward Arnold, Sevenoaks

Saunders C (1999) Comments made during European Association for Palliative Care 6th Conference, Geneva, Switzerland

Sheldon F (1997) *Psychosocial Palliative Care.* Stanley Thornes, Cheltenham

Walter T (1996) A new model of grief: bereavement and biography. *Mortality* **1**(1): 7–25

Walter T (1999) *On Bereavement: the Culture of Grief.* Open University Press, Buckinghamshire

Weinstein J, Whittington C, Leiba T (eds) (2003) *Collaboration in Social Work Practice.* Jessica Kingsley, London

Whittington C (2003a) *Learning for Collaborative Practice.* DoH, London

Whittington C (2003b) Collaboration and partnership in context. In: Weinstein J, Whittington C, Leiba T (eds) *Collaboration in Social Work Practice.* Jessica Kingsley, London

Chapter 5

Social work and bereavement support — a perspective from palliative care

Barbara Parker

Introduction

In this chapter, the complexities of bereavement and the grieving process will be introduced. I will also explore the more mundane and practical aspects of the loss of a loved one. Death affects us all in different ways; this chapter does not attempt to tell anybody how they should or should not grieve. It acknowledges that cultural, individual and historical factors affect our responses. The chapter is written in relation to contemporary UK society, and explores the role of palliative care social work within bereavement services. I will begin by examining some of the terms that are used in this field.

Definitions: 'bereavement', 'grief' and 'mourning'

The words 'bereavement', 'grief' and 'mourning' are often used without question and it is valuable to explore what these terms mean before we consider some of the theories developed to expound them.

According to Payne *et al* (1999), 'bereavement' and 'grief' have a common root: the Old English word 'reafian' which means to plunder, spoil or rob. The root meaning denotes a sudden and forceful deprivation. They also suggest that the words imply an emotional attachment to the lost object: 'These two aspects of loss by death — the sense of personal violation and the heaviness of the soul — are thus embedded in the language itself' (Payne *et al*, 1999: 6).

Although both 'bereavement' and 'grief' have the same root, there are differences in the definition and in the uses of these two terms. Stroebe and Schut (1998: 7) provide a fairly simple definition of 'bereavement': 'the situation of a person who has recently experienced the loss of someone significant through that person's death'. Dershimer (1990: 17), moreover, includes not only the 'situation' but also the 'process' in his understanding of the word:

> *Bereavement... describes the total recovery process of humans from the death of someone with whom they had a significant relationship. Bereavement includes much more than the pain of grief. It includes significant changes in the behaviour, thoughts, attitudes, and in the religious and spiritual life of the bereaved... Grief does not simply come and go. It must be dealt with, and because it is profoundly complicated, it calls upon individuals to make fundamental changes in their lives. That process is called 'bereavement'.*

Rather than including the process in their definition of 'bereavement', as Dershimer does, most authors suggest that process is inherent in the term 'grief'. Parkes (1996: 7) writes: 'Grief is a process, not a state. It is the reaction to a loss, usually of a person'. Faulberg (cited in Currer, 2001: 91) takes it one step further by describing 'grief' not only as a reaction to loss, but also as 'the process through which one passes in order to recover from loss'. Martin and Doka (2000: 16) describe 'grief' as 'an emotion, an attempt to make internal and external adjustments to the undesired change in one's world brought about by loss'. Here, 'grief' encompasses the idea of process, together with ideas of adjustment and recovery.

'Mourning', although associated with grief and bereavement, has a slightly different meaning; it has a cultural or societal basis. Stroebe and Schut (1998: 7) write: 'mourning refers to the social expressions of grief, which are shaped by the practice of a given society or cultural group'. Martin and Doka (2000) also suggest that 'mourning' is culturally and socially based, and that the rituals involved allow others to recognise that the individual has been bereaved.

In summary, there are, in the literature, some succinct definitions that give clear distinctions between these three words, bereavement, grief and mourning. Oliviere *et al* (1998: 121) encapsulate this well: 'bereavement is an event; grief is the emotional process; mourning is the cultural process.' Stroebe *et al* (1993: 5) write: 'bereavement is the objective situation of having lost someone significant; grief is the emotional response to one's loss; and mourning denotes the actions and manner of expressing grief, which often reflect the mourning practices of one's culture.' On the face of it, these two definitions appear to be the same, or at least very similar. However, as Payne and Lloyd-Williams (2003: 151) suggest, how we define bereavement has a bearing on our understanding of the bereavement experience itself. For the purposes of this chapter, I will work with the definition given by Stroebe *et al* (1993) because they move away from the idea of process and recovery and encompass a wider range of models within their definition.

One further point: although definitions of bereavement and grief generally concern the individual affected by the loss, and mourning concerns the social and cultural contexts, the experience of loss does not occur in isolation — it takes place in the context of family, society and culture. Social workers are concerned with well-being in this wider context, and must take these dimensions into account when working with people who are bereaved. As we shall see, this wider context has implications for the theories that have been developed to understand bereavement and grieving, and to promote the development of systemic, multidimensional approaches.

Models and theories of grief and bereavement

Models and theories of grief have developed over time, and will continue to develop. Each of the models has something to contribute to our growing understanding of bereavement and grief, and it is therefore important that we consider them. Since it is impossible to give a detailed account of them all here, I will concentrate on providing broad overviews of:

- grief as a 'process'
- continuity theories
- grief related to stress and coping styles
- the family context of grief.

Early theories and grief as a 'process'

It was Sigmund Freud, in *Mourning and Melancholia* (1917), who first differentiated grieving from depression. Freud stated that grieving presents the individual with a difficulty because they need to relinquish the relationship with the deceased to regain the emotional energy invested, but the individual also wishes to maintain a bond with, and somehow 'hold on to', the loved object.

Bowlby and Parkes have had a major influence on the development of process models. Bowlby's attachment theory postulates that early in life we all form affectional bonds and that these early attachments influence our relationships throughout life. Formation, disruption and maintenance of attachment bonds give rise to intense emotions. Loss of the attachment figure leads to grief (see Currer, 2001). Bowlby (1980: 93) argues that working through the phases of grief is a necessary aspect of 'successful' mourning.

Kübler-Ross's (1969) famous 'stages' are often applied to those who are bereaved. Undertaking clinical work as a psychiatrist, Kübler-Ross was able to identify the reactions of dying patients and from this identified 'stages of dying'. She argued that often the initial reaction was one of denial and isolation, which was a way for individuals to manage shock and take in the news. Once the patient begins to accept the diagnosis, anger sets in — towards self or others. Bargaining, often with God, and usually related to cure, was the next reaction that she identified. When bargaining is seen as not working, and the truth of the impending death becomes more real, depression sets in, together with feelings of sadness and overwhelming loss. The final stage, according to Kübler-Ross, is acceptance, as the reality of the impending death is absorbed, followed by peacefulness.

Although Kübler-Ross's model can be useful in considering the process of bereavement, she never intended these ideas to be applied to bereavement. She also acknowledged that not everyone who is dying will go through all these stages or experience them in this order.

Parkes's understanding of grief has changed and developed through the three editions of his book, *Bereavement: Studies of Grief in Adult Life*. In the first edition, he identifies four phases in the grief process, which are very similar to those put forward by Bowlby:

1. Numbness, shock, disbelief.
2. Yearning or searching.
3. Disorganisation and despair.
4. Recovery.

He intended that these phases would be recognised as overlapping, and that individual experiences of grief would vary. In the second edition, Parkes writes: 'grief is a process and not a state. Grief is not a set of symptoms which start after a loss and then gradually fade away. It involves a succession of clinical pictures which blend into and replace one another'. Importantly, in the third edition (1996), and in addition to the phase model, Parkes also explores the idea of bereavement as a psychosocial transition, perhaps recognising the limitations of the phase model when used in isolation.

Worden (1991) proposes that since grief is a process, people need to work through their reactions to make a complete adjustment. He identifies four tasks of mourning which, as Payne *et al* (1999: 74) acknowledge, have been 'extremely influential and widely used by those working with bereaved people':

Task 1. To accept the reality of the loss.
Task 2. To work through the pain of the grief.
Task 3. To adjust to the environment without the deceased.
Task 4. To emotionally relocate the deceased and move on with life.

Originally, the fourth task outlined the need to detach and form new relationships. Worden (1991: 16) revised this task in his second edition because he believed it had been misunderstood. As in the previous phase and stage models, Worden's tasks were not intended to be prescriptive; instead, they were to encapsulate the idea that the individual is not merely passive in the situation of grief, but that he or she can actively alter and move towards change.

Even though each of the process models stressed the fluidity of the stages, phases or tasks, there has always been a tendency to view them as prescriptive and linear. There is also a danger that they will be misinterpreted in being used to define 'how' bereaved people should respond (Payne *et al*, 1999). This is clearly not their purpose and there is sufficient research to show that they do not function in this way (Stroebe *et al*, 1993). There have also been criticisms that the process models are so prescriptive that they do not take into account cultural and gender differences in grieving (see Currer, 2001: 98). The process models have also been taken to indicate that the final stage of grief is 'recovery', which has been questioned by Klass *et al*'s (1996) idea of 'continuing bonds', which will be discussed in the next section. Payne *et al* (1999: 83) write:

> *the general consensus is that phase models provide useful descriptions of the course of grief and can be of great value as a general guide for both professionals and lay people, helping them to understand common grief experiences. However, they may need to be augmented by other models.*

Continuity theories

In the mid-to-late 1990s, bereavement models began to move away from the idea of process and recovery. There are a number of reasons why this happened, including the fact that many bereaved people felt that the process models did not do justice to their experience and also that research began to indicate that there are cultural and gender differences in grieving, for which established models made no space (Stroebe, 1998; Stroebe and Schut, 1998).

Klass *et al* (1996) suggest that the deceased may continue to influence the lives of the bereaved without problems occurring. Memories of the deceased, the impact they made on individual lives, incorporating the deceased's ideas and values, and continuing the work of the deceased — all are recognised and acknowledged as being within the normal boundaries of bereavement behaviour. Klass *et al* (1996: 19) also suggest that far from 'detaching' from the deceased, those surviving move into a different relationship with them. The purpose of grief is not to detach and forget, but to relocate and remember:

> *The studies in this book suggest that we need to consider bereavement as a cognitive as well as an emotional process that takes place in a social context of which the deceased is a part. The process does not end, but in different ways bereavement affects the mourner for the rest of his or her life. People are changed by the experience; they do not get over it, and part of the change is a transformed but continuing relationship with the deceased.*

Walter (1996: 13–14), writing from a sociological perspective, asks us to focus bereavement work on biography rather than feelings. He states that the purpose of grief is to find a secure place in our lives for the person who has died, and that we need to do this through biography. He suggests that this is better if it's a shared biography. Grieving encompasses the task of:

> *jointly constructing an accurate picture of the dead person... It is... important for survivors that they can piece together how this person affected their own lives.*

This is to do with establishing purpose, meaning and making sense of life. However, Walter acknowledges that creating a shared narrative can be hindered by the circumstances common to modern life: geographical mobility, longevity, lack of community, separation of work and home life, and so on. He states that talking about feelings to an outsider is 'a poor second best' (1996: 19) and that talking to others who knew the deceased is preferable.

The acknowledgement of continuing relationships and subjective responses fits well with social work's acknowledgement of diversity. However, we must acknowledge some criticisms of this understanding.

'Continuing bonds' suggests that an ongoing relationship with the deceased is a healthy component of grief — yet where is the evidence? Gal-Oz and Field (2002) suggest that the empirical evidence is limited. In their research, they found that the relation between connections maintained with the deceased and adjustment to bereavement is complex, indicating that not all expressions of a continuing bond are helpful in the constructive resolution of grief. They go on to argue that their research has implications for bereavement support:

> *It is important for bereavement counsellors to be able to distinguish between a continuing bond which is an attempt to deny reality and one which is a healthy expression of the positive impact of the deceased carried forward into the new life of the bereaved.*

> (Gal-Oz and Field, 2002: 43)

The main criticism of Walter's idea is that the research-base is weak, based (critics claim) on personal rather than common (or universal) experience. Walter suggests that bereavement is about biography rather than feelings, but can feelings be ignored when we consider the impact and strength of the feelings experienced? Indeed, Stroebe (1997) points out that working through feelings and integrating the meaning of the relationship are connected, rather than separate, processes.

The continuity models explored here emphasise the interpersonal and social context of grieving. The models have created more emphasis on encouraging the bereaved to tell their story in the therapeutic setting, rather than just concentrating on feelings. They acknowledge the need for the bereaved to have information — going over the last chapter with doctors and nurses has some validity and purpose. This has had a profound effect on the way funerals are carried out. It is now accepted that the individual's life-story is of prime importance to the funeral. The continuity models, because they explore the ongoing relationship with the deceased, also encompass the need to create meaning from the experience of bereavement.

Grief related to stress and coping styles

In looking at the literature on grief and bereavement, we need to look at stress and coping. 'Stress models of grief consider bereavement as a stressful life event and offer an explanation for the physical health consequences of bereavement' (Stroebe *et al*, 1993: 7).

The dual-process model (Stroebe and Schut, 1999) suggests that there are two categories of stressor in bereavement:

1. Coping with the loss itself.
2. Coping with other changes and adjustments that result from it.

Stroebe and Schut (1999) suggest that people undertake in varying proportions (according to individual and cultural variations) what they call loss-orientated and restoration-orientated coping.

Loss-orientation concerns some aspect of the loss experience itself, especially with respect to the deceased person. It may involve ruminating about that person, about life together, the circumstances and events around the death itself; and also yearning for the deceased, looking at photographs, and crying about the death. A range of emotions are involved, from distress and pain to pleasure (in memories) and relief (that the deceased is no longer suffering).

Restoration-orientation refers to what needs to be dealt with, and how. This includes mastering the tasks that the deceased undertook; dealing with the arrangements for the reorganisation of life without the deceased; developing a new identity from 'wife' to 'widow'; and so on.

These two forms of orientation are summed up well by Stroebe and Schut (1999: 206):

> *when a loved one dies, not only is there grief for the deceased*
> *person, one also has to adjust to substantial changes that are*
> *secondary consequences to the loss.*

The central component of the model is 'oscillation' — that is, the individual needs to move between the orientations, alternating between loss-orientation and restoration-orientation to grieve in a healthy manner. The individual takes time out from the emotional distress of the grief to deal with everyday life; in

Stroebe and Schut's words (1999: 209), the pain of the grieving 'needs dosage'. In the model, it is suggested that one of the orientations may predominate according to culture, gender and the circumstances of the death. It is also suggested that in the broader context, behaviour is likely to shift over time from loss-orientation to restoration-orientation.

Similarly, Martin and Doka's (2000) model relates bereavement responses to coping styles. They identified two styles of response in bereavement: the instrumental response and the intuitive response. In the intuitive pattern, there is an emphasis on effect, the emotional response to bereavement, and the person who grieves in this way gains strength from sharing and expressing feelings. In the instrumental pattern, however, there is an emphasis on cognition, and thinking often takes precedence over, and precedes, feelings. The instrumental griever is reluctant to talk about feelings and prefers problem-solving strategies. For instrumental grievers, activity helps with adjustment. Activity is often used as a way of memorialising the deceased: carving an urn, digging a grave, planting a tree. Solving problems associated with the loss often gives the griever an effective outlet for action: taking over the business, joining or creating an organisation promoting a cause associated with the death, or making restitution for any damage caused or injury in the wake of the death. Activity can also restore normalcy, a sense of security — returning to school or to work. Martin and Doka suggest that the two patterns of grieving lie at opposite ends of a continuum, and that most people have, to a greater or lesser degree, a 'blended' style of grieving: although one style is likely to be dominant, there will generally be a mixture.

These 'coping styles' models have some areas of difficulty. They do not, for example, explain the role of interpersonal relationships in helping people cope with loss. Also, there is no recognition that the search for meaning has a place in bereavement behaviours. With Martin and Doka's model, there is a danger of gender stereotyping, despite the fact that they warn against it.

However, the 'coping styles' do provide clear guidelines for those working with the bereaved, and their strength is in giving credence to individual ways of coping with loss.

Family context of grieving models

Rosenblatt (1993: 102), in his family systems theory, emphasises how family rules and patterns shape loss experiences and how a significant loss affects and is played out in a system of family relationships. He suggests that the family, when a death occurs, loses its structure and hence its ability to support the individuals within that structure (1993: 103). Thus, the grief for the person who has died 'may be compounded by grieving for the system that now seems inadequate to meet the survivors' needs' (1993: 106). Following on from this, he suggests that within the grieving family, arguments occur together with anger and blame directed at one another (1993: 106).

Worden (1991) also recognises the importance of the family system. He suggests that maintaining balance in the family is vital: 'most families exist in some type of homeostatic balance, and the loss of a significant person in that family group can unbalance this homeostasis and cause the family to feel pain and seek help' (1991: 149). He suggests there are three areas that need to be considered when assessing how a family will continue to function following a death: first, whether the deceased played a significant role within the family; second, whether the family is emotionally integrated and hence able to support one another; and third, whether the family are able to help one another express themselves emotionally (1991: 150–2).

This leads us to consider the multiple dimensions of grief. There is general recognition that grief is multi-faceted, but there are several investigators whose models are specifically around the multiple dimensional nature of grief. Susan Le Poidevin's seven dimensions of grief (referred to in Payne *et al*, 1999: 84) can be helpful, as can Schuter and Zisook's six dimensions (cited by Payne *et al*, 1999: 85). These draw attention to the fact that grief has many different aspects and that coping with the emotional and cognitive responses and pain — as well as making adjustments in relationships, functioning and identity — are an essential part of grief.

In considering family grieving, it is important to remember that families exist in many different forms. Although most individuals exist as part of a family group, the family is not necessarily supportive or helpful when bereavement occurs. But it is central that the social worker has an understanding of the person in context in order to consider appropriate means of support. The multidimensional models are helpful to the social worker in providing an understanding of the wider framework in which the individual exists, and hence for which the individual may gain support. These models also help to prevent grief being seem as static or linear.

Reasons why theories exist

Theories and models help us understand reactions and symptoms; they provide explanations for individual differences and from them strategies can be devised as how best to help people. However, no one theory fulfils all of these all of the time, as Lloyd-Williams ([ed], 2003: 149) recognises:

It is generally agreed that there are no single 'correct' or 'true' theories that explain the experience of loss or account for the emotions, experiences and cultural practices which characterise grief and mourning.

It is clear that individuals react differently to loss, and that the diversity of models contributes to the social worker's understanding and therefore range of interventive techniques that can be used.

Case study

Jane is the bereaved partner of Mary. Mary died recently in the hospice following a relatively short illness. She and Jane met following the breakdown of Mary's marriage. They set up home together two years ago. Mary's family never accepted the relationship; they always referred to Jane as Mary's 'friend' or 'housemate'. During her illness, there was some animosity towards Jane from Mary's parents and her ex-husband, but Jane continued to care for her and encouraged the family to visit until her admission to the hospice. Since her death, Mary's family have 'taken charge'. They refused to allow Jane to attend the funeral and have demanded that Jane return all Mary's possessions to them.

This case study will be referred to in the rest of this chapter, along with other examples of practice.

How does the social worker use bereavement theories and models in palliative care?

Having considered the bereavement theories and models and, briefly, critiqued them, we must now ask how they are appropriate to the social worker in palliative care. Clearly, they are useful in direct work with the bereaved, but they also have a relevance to interdisciplinary working and an impact on the planning and development of the bereavement services provided by the hospice or palliative-care setting (see *Chapter 6* and *Chapter 4*). We will consider three core areas in which models and theories are used:

A. With service users.
B. Within the inter-disciplinary setting.
C. Structuring services.

A. With service users

1. Normalising the experience of grief

Bereavement literature serves to normalise the experience of grief. Some of the behaviours resulting from bereavement could be regarded as bizarre, but in the context of such loss, they are 'to be expected'. For example, the process models suggest that there is a recognised pattern to grieving and that this process begins with a period of denial, followed by a period of searching behaviour. So when a bereaved person is worried that, although they know that the person has died, they expect to hear him come home at a certain time — or think, 'I must tell him such and such' — finding out from their social worker that such experiences are part of the normal process of grieving, the individual feels reassured that he or she is not 'going mad'.

There are countless further examples. A gentleman recently came to see me, concerned that he was generally a 'laid-back' person, but that since his father's death he had become extremely short-tempered. Again, this is a very normal reaction following the death of someone close, and having been given this reassurance, he felt better able to deal with it.

In relation to the case study, for example, Jane might feel the need to sleep with Mary's nightdress because it gives her a feeling of 'nearness' to Mary. To the outside world, this might seem bizarre, but the social worker could assure Jane that this is normal behaviour in the context of bereavement.

The Dual Process Model (Stroebe and Schut, 1999) suggests that it is acceptable (or 'okay') to 'take time off from the grief', and that both controlling feelings and expressing them are important. Again, if reassurance can be given that this is the norm, the individual will be better able to deal with it and accept it. Indeed, Martin and Doka (2000) suggest that instrumental grievers are often reluctant to talk about their feelings. We are in an age where 'it's good to talk' is frequently seen as a philosophy of life, and often other family members are worried if an individual does not feel the need to talk. Statements such as, 'He's bottling it all up' and 'He really needs to talk' are common — but not necessarily true. The social worker can reassure family members by telling them that it is not necessarily 'good to talk', as many researchers recognise.

For example, a mother and her adult daughter came to see me. The mother was worried that her daughter was not talking about the death of her father or expressing any emotions. During the interview, it became clear that the daughter didn't feel the need to talk, but that she was putting together a photograph album of her father which she would remember him by. I was able to explain Martin and Doka's theory about instrumental grievers to both of them. The mother was clearly relieved to find an explanation for her daughter's behaviour.

2. Information and education

The social worker's role with the bereaved is one of information and education. Generally, individuals cope better with any crisis if they are given sufficient relevant information — this is also true of bereavement. The social worker can provide general written information that is available to all — for example, at Dove House Hospice, we have a *Bereavement Information Booklet* that contains information about feelings, thoughts and other reactions to loss.

This information is guided by the current theories and models. In specific situations, it is appropriate for the social worker to educate the service user regarding a specific model that may provide helpful information to the bereaved person. I have recently used the Dual Purpose Model with one service user to review their progress. I also used it to help suggest to another bereaved person that she was so busy getting on with the practical changes and adapting to life without her partner that she was not allowing herself to examine the loss and experience its full emotional impact. The idea of oscillation proved helpful to this lady because she was able to see that she didn't need to 'give up' the adjustment side completely — just move between the two approaches. This allowed her to see that it would be 'safe' to explore her feelings and thoughts because she would be able to return to adjustment afterwards.

The other important reason for 'educating' the bereaved is that it helps prevent misconceptions about what is right and expected. The common understanding of grieving is that it comes to an end. But statements such as 'we have closure' or 'you'll get over it' are very unhelpful to those who are grieving. If the social worker is able to inform the individual that the continuity models allow for the continuing relationship with the deceased, then once again they can be reassured that their behaviour is within normal boundaries.

3. Interventions with service users

Specific interventions with the bereaved follow on from bereavement models.

(a) Exploring feelings: For many people, this is very important at the onset of bereavement intervention as they may be overwhelmed by feelings of grief. Some of these feelings are totally unexpected and will need to be carefully explored, encouraging the individual to express what they are experiencing. Counselling skills are useful for the social worker in helping the individual express themselves (see *Chapter 6*). The need to explore feelings can be seen if we base our intervention on the various process models and specifically if we use Worden's first task — to feel the pain. Martin and Doka suggest that the intuitive griever has a need to express feelings to others. It may be that by involving the bereaved in a support group, where they meet others in similar

situations, they are given the opportunity to explore and express their feelings. Groups can also be beneficial in 'normalising' the grief experience, in that behaviours, thoughts and feelings can be expressed and 'checked out' against other people's experiences.

At a meeting of a group at my hospice some time ago, one of the gentlemen, who up until that point had made very little contribution to the group, hesitantly asked if he could share something with the group. He went on to talk about some 'strange' things that had been happening to him in the weeks following his wife's death — a clock had stopped at the time of death; a soft toy, which she had had from childhood, had fallen off a shelf; and so on. At this point, each member of the group was able to open up and tell their own story of 'strange' happenings, and a discussion took place that took the group into issues about life after death, the 'spirit world', and distinguishing between hopes and realities. They clearly felt comfortable discussing these issues within the group situation, mainly because it served to normalise their own experiences.

(b) Telling the story: If we look at Walter's ideas, it is clear that there is a need for the bereaved person to 'create a shared biography'. The social worker can encourage the individual to enter into social situations where there would be the opportunity to share with those who knew the deceased — for example, to attend the funeral or the funeral tea, or even to encourage the bereaved to create a social situation where this might be possible, as in a friends' get-together. It may be that the social worker would help the individual identify who might be appropriate to share the story with. This could be done by the use of an ecomap or 'caring circles' where family and friends are identified and then placed within a system to enable recognition of who is most likely to be able to provide what the individual needs (see *Figure 5.1*). If we consider the case study earlier, we may see that Mary's family would have a contribution to make in forming a 'shared biography' with Jane (ie. be able to share parts of Mary's life previously unknown to Jane). However, it is also clear that because of their reluctance to accept Jane as Mary's partner, it is unlikely that they would be willing to share in a positive way. The social worker might encourage

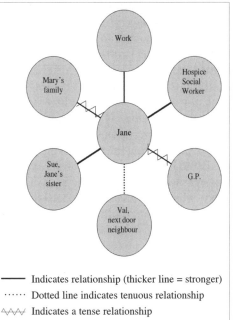

—— Indicates relationship (thicker line = stronger)
······ Dotted line indicates tenuous relationship
∿∿∿ Indicates a tense relationship

Figure 5.1: An ecomap showing Jane's support network

Jane to seek out friends or work colleagues with whom she could draw together some sort of biography or simply reminisce.

It is often valid for the social worker to enter into a 'biography construction' with the bereaved — for example, if there are no family and friends to create a shared biography with, as may well be the case for Jane. It is also useful to use biography if the individual finds it too painful or personal to talk about feelings; telling the story can be a fairly safe starting point. It clarifies for the bereaved what actually happened; it helps the social worker understand the bereavement in its context; and it helps to identify any actual or potential difficulties. It can be difficult to get someone started, but I have found that a simple statement or question is usually sufficient. 'Tell me about your husband' will often elicit the response, 'where do you want me to start?' which can then be followed by 'had he been ill for long?' With encouraging remarks and the use of other listening skills, the story wll then generally follow. In these early interviews, it is not essential to get a blow-by-blow account or necessarily to have events recounted in the right order, but more to allow the individual to explore the period of illness, its ups and downs, its hopes and 'if only's. It may be through telling the story that practical issues come to light which need to be addressed, such as complaints about the care the deceased received; issues with the GP; or indeed with your own service.

*(c) **Memorialising the deceased***: In Martin and Doka's ideas about the instrumental pattern of grieving, there is a different type of intervention that involves encouraging or enabling the memorialisation of the deceased. The social worker's role here can be to help the individual explore the different options and to make decisions in line with their own needs. The funeral provides an immediate and expected occurrence where the deceased will be memorialised. From this, there are a number of associated options for memorialising, such as choosing a headstone or making decisions about where to place ashes following cremation, together with decisions about, say, planting rose trees in the local crematorium or creating a special garden at home.

In considering memorialising the deceased, it is important for the social worker to be aware of, and sensitive to, cultural differences and to explore options appropriate to cultural practices. The social worker can provide information about what is available and help the individual explore how best to meet their own personal and cultural needs and those of the wider family and friends in creating specific memorials for the deceased. It may be that several weeks after the death, the individual could attend or create a memorial service for the deceased. Memorialisation does not necessarily need to be formal, compiling an album of photographs or creating a 'memory box' are excellent ways of creating a memorial. Other methods of memorialisation might include joining or creating an organisation in some way related to the death; setting up a website; campaigning for better services; raising public awareness about certain diseases; becoming involved in raising funds for new equipment or to support existing services; and volunteering in a specific organisation. Traditionally, we have tended to encourage people to hold back from these types of activities until they have reached some sort of stability. It seems, however, from Martin and Doka's ideas that, for some people, stability will not be achieved until they have entered into these memorialising tasks. For those who grieve in a largely instrumental way, these acts of memorialising are key to achieving adjustment to the loss.

In Jane's situation, as she has not been allowed to attend the funeral, the social worker may enable her to consider other options for memorialising. She could hold a memorial service for Mary, open to family and friends at a local venue, be it a place of religious worship or a place that was special to them both. She may decide to create a memorial in a public or private place — for example, she could place Mary's name in a book of remembrance at the hospice where she died, plant a rose tree in the garden at home, or create a scrapbook of letters she wrote. Exploring the options available to Jane after Mary's death could be a key part of the social worker's supportive role.

(d) Learning new skills: If we look at the Dual Process Model (Stroebe and Schut, 1999), there is a clear need within restoration-orientation to tackle some of the practical issues; in doing so, new skills are learned. In terms of practical tasks, there are both major and minor things to be done. In this section, I will discuss the minor tasks (the major tasks are briefly discussed in the next section).

The business of getting on with day to day life has to be addressed fairly soon in bereavement. In any partnership, the tasks of everyday life are shared between the partners. If a partner dies, the tasks fall to the surviving individual. Some things may appear daunting to the newly bereaved. For example, a lady whose husband took care of the cars now had to take responsibility for this herself. She was anxious about how to put petrol in the car and decided to overcome this difficulty by asking her son-in-law if he would accompany her on her first visit to the garage and teach her.

In her recent book about her life with the English actor John Thaw (famous for his role as TV's *Inspector Morse*, among others), Sheila Hancock (2004: 223) writes that after he had died:

> one of the crew of Bedtime *said, 'Your tyres are worn out and dangerous, Sheila.' I didn't know what to do. John would have dealt with these things. But I got it sorted. I've bloody well got to learn to cope. Felt quite pleased with myself.*

Not only are there new tasks to learn, then, but completing them successfully can create a sense of achievement at a time when the bereaved feels overwhelmed by their new responsibilities. Those supporting the bereaved may find it helpful to use the new achievements to encourage the bereaved to tackle other equally daunting new tasks. By direct referral to the Dual Process Model, and perhaps even using drawings as a visual aid, the social worker may be able to show the bereaved that the two forms of loss, loss-orientation and restoration-orientation, are vital for adjustment.

(e) 'Sorting out the mess': Not only are there new small tasks to be completed, but the bereaved might also have to address much bigger issues. Initially, there are decisions that need to made about the funeral; then there is the question of how to pay for the funeral. There is the deceased's estate to deal with, which may involve wills and probate and involve solicitors. There are decisions to be made with regard to disposal of the deceased's possessions. Often people seek reassurance that what they are doing is 'right' and have to balance the conflicting advice of various family members. There may be decisions to make about the deceased's business — whether to wind it up or continue to run it. There may be issues around the future care of children, housing and finances. There may be complaints about the care received by the deceased during the illness, or family disputes that need to be reconciled.

In Jane's situation, she has been cut out of the funeral and the mourning practices of the family members, who have also made demands on her regarding Mary's possessions. The social worker may be required to help Jane seek legal advice in this situation. Jane may decide to negotiate with the family about possessions and may need support from the social worker as the disputes take place, or may indeed wish the social worker to take on the role of intermediary. It may be that Jane is made homeless by the situation and may need some help negotiating the various housing authorities to consider her options. Bereavement not only creates difficult emotional hurdles; it can also have profound practical consequences.

(f) Moving forwards: There is little written about the long-terms effects of bereavement, with a general view that after about two years, adjustment to the new situation will normally have taken place. Moving forwards has its own difficulties. Individuals can often feel as though they are betraying the deceased by taking control of their lives again; families may object to the way in which a person moves forward (for example, if they become involved in a new relationship). Again, the social worker may need to use skills of normalisation to help families achieve good communication at this time. It is key to recognise that there is no 'right way' of moving forwards and that each individual, according to his or her circumstances, needs to find their own way through these difficulties. This brings us to the question of complicated grieving: when should we worry about the way we are grieving? There are several useful guidelines — for details, see Worden (2003), chapters 4 and 5, and Stroebe *et al* (1993), chapters 3 and 18.

B. Within the interdisciplinary setting

1. An educational role

Within the interdisciplinary setting of any palliative care service, there are several different professionals working alongside one another. There is a need to understand each individual's role within this setting and to understand the expertise contained within this team (see *Chapter 4*). A basic understanding of bereavement is essential in creating an atmosphere that aims to elicit a good bereavement outcome. Implicit in the care of the dying is the need to care for the survivors. As with any education or training, there is also a need for regular updating of information with regard to bereavement theories and interventions. The social worker working within bereavement support will be best placed to offer up-to-date, in-house education and training, be it formal or informal, within the inter-disciplinary setting.

2. An integrated role

Bereavement services are clearly an essential part of the overall services offered in hospice and other palliative care settings. The NICE guidelines recognise that the care offered to relatives and friends both during the illness and after death is essential (NHS, 2004). Oliviere *et al* (1998) argue that the bereavement services need to be integrated into the general palliative care services provided, rather than being a 'bolt on' at the end. Indeed, from recent research (Field *et al*, 2003: 2), it is clear that the bereavement services are seen as integral by the hospices themselves:

> *The modern hospice movement has recognised the continuing needs of the bereaved relatives of their patients… and most hospices now regard the provision of such support as an integral part of their services.*

During a recent meeting of the North East and Yorkshire regional meeting of Bereavement Service Coordinators, I asked if the participants believed that the bereavement services were well integrated into their particular setting. The vast majority said that they were. On further exploration, it was clear that integration occurred because of the following main factors:

a.   Being recognised as part of the multidisciplinary team, including attending multidisciplinary meetings.

b. Working alongside, and doing joint work with, colleagues who are not part of the bereavement team.
c. Being actively involved in pre-bereavement support.
d. Being involved in the training and teaching of other professionals about the work of the bereavement service.

Each of these factors reflects the need to work alongside other professionals and disciplines as an essential aspect of integration. Oliviere *et al* (1998: 139–40) make this point:

It is essential to attempt to integrate the bereavement service with the total palliative service, so that it does not become the exclusive property of those running it — shared ownership is part of its success.

I believe, however, that there is more that can be done to create greater recognition for bereavement services. Field *et al* (2003: 12) note that:

Adult bereavement services are relatively small, typically involving two to three paid staff, not all of whom are necessarily working full-time for the service. The staff primarily involved in running the services usually hold a qualification in nursing, counselling or social work. Both the small size of the bereavement support services and the predominance of staff who are not seen as centrally involved in clinical decision-making suggest that, despite the rhetoric that it is integral to hospice and specialist palliative care services, in practice, adult bereavement support remains marginal to the core activities of patient care.

This view is echoed is by Lloyd-Williams (2003) when she writes that bereavement services usually involve nurses and social workers, but that medical staff, who are usually involved in other aspects of specialist palliative care services, are often not involved in the bereavement services. The conclusion is that bereavement services could be better integrated into the work of the hospice or specialist palliative care setting.

C. Structuring services

The NICE guidelines suggest a three-component model of bereavement support (NHS, 2004: 161):

⌘ **Component 1**: First of all, the fact that not everyone needs bereavement support is recognised, but it is recommended that everyone has access to information about the experience of grief and how to access support if needed.

⌘ **Component 2**: The guidelines suggest that some people will need a 'more formal opportunity to review and reflect on their loss experience' and that a service of this nature does not necessarily need to be provided by professionals but can be provided by volunteer bereavement support workers, self-help groups and others.

⌘ **Component 3**: Some people will need more specialist interventions such as from mental health services, or help from counsellors or specialist bereavement services, and these should be accessible to those who require specialist interventions.

The guidelines also suggest that the bereavement services need to provide support for staff who are continually experiencing loss because of the nature of their work — this would include nursing staff, ancillary workers who have patient contact, and medical staff. It is also recognised that further research is needed to compare different models of bereavement support and to determine in which situation and for which individuals support is needed. The guidelines suggest that screening needs to be in place to assess levels of vulnerability.

Ideally, bereavement services would be structured to meet each of the components referred to in the NICE guidelines. Assessment needs to be in place so that those who are bereaved can be screened to gauge their level of vulnerability and to direct appropriate services to individual needs. However, there is no single assessment method that has a large degree of reliability, so this is clearly an area that warrants further research (see Payne and Relf, 1994; Field *et al*, 2004: 575).

In the meantime, we are left creating services that we feel will best meet our service users' needs. If we base our bereavement services on the theories and models, we stand a chance of achieving that goal. First of all, services need to be accessible and flexible, and the greater the menu of services offered the more likely we are to be catering for the needs of people. Services should include information about the experience of grief and the support available. The support services need to offer the opportunity to talk about feelings and about the 'story', whether this is in groups or one-to-one. Family support needs to be included if we are to reflect adequately the social situation in which many deaths take place, and the emphasis of some of the models on family interactions.

There also needs to be a memorial dimension to the services offered. The hospice may offer a memorial event where all the bereaved are invited. There may be opportunities to create specific individual memorial events — planting specific flowers in the hospice grounds, or purchasing a leaf for a memorial tree, or a stone for a memorial garden. Acts of memorial demand creativity and cultural sensitivity, and need to be in keeping with the desire of the bereaved to memorialise. Any bereavement service must be flexible enough to be able to address individual need, whether there are practical issues, financial difficulties, social problems, spiritual issues or cultural needs, and each of these factors needs to be borne in mind when developing any bereavement service.

The bereavement service at Dove House aims to reflect the diversity of the needs of the bereaved. Information about the practical issues that need to be addressed is given shortly after the death. After several weeks, the family will receive a booklet that contains information about the experience of grief. At eight to twelve weeks after the death, a bereavement support worker will make telephone contact to give information about the support available and also to make an assessment of the individual's needs. A variety of support is available. The individual can choose to receive weekly or fortnightly supportive telephone contact; they can receive face to face individual counselling or support; or they can attend a support group. Each family is also offered the opportunity to attend an 'Afternoon for Remembering', which is a memorial event available to all. If there are specific difficulties, such as financial or legal issues, or a clear indication of lengthy support being needed, the family or individual will be offered professional support through the social work team.

There is, however, much to do. We eagerly await the development of a reliable risk-assessment tool, but, in the meantime, we often use clinical judgement to decide when to offer support. We need to consider developing a more formal approach to supporting families as a whole, rather than as individuals. We need to seek more diversity in the ways by which we encourage memorialising those who have died. Furthermore, there is a responsibility for bereavement services to offer support to staff, which is something we need to develop within Dove House.

Conclusion

In this chapter, I have examined the theories and models of bereavement and their impact on, and implications for, social workers working within bereavement services. The implications of using models and frameworks for practice relate not only to the interventions undertaken with the service-user, but also to the position of the bereavement services within the specific palliative care setting; they have a bearing, as well, on how these services are structured. This chapter has considered best practice in terms of each of these areas. Just as our understanding and knowledge of bereavement will continue to grow and develop as research into new ideas and models accumulates, so bereavement services also need to develop to continue providing an effective service.

References

Bowlby J (1980) *Attachment and Loss, Vol 3: Loss — Sadness and Depression.* Hogarth Press, London

Currer C (2001) *Responding to Grief: Dying, Bereavement and Social Care.* Palgrave, Basingstoke

Dershimer RA (1990) *Counselling the Bereaved.* Pergamon Press, Oxford

Field D, Reid D, Payne S, Relf M (2003) *A National Postal Survey of Adult Bereavement Services in Hospice and Specialist Palliative Care Services in the UK, 2003: Report to the Respondents.* Sheffield: Palliative and End-of-Life Care Research Group, University of Sheffield

Field D, Reid D, Payne S, Relf M (2004) Survey of UK hospice and specialist palliative care adult bereavement services. *Int J Palliat Nurs* **10**(12): 569–76

Freud S (1917) *Mourning and Melancholia, Collected Papers, 4.* Basic Books, New York

Gal-Oz E, Field N (2002) Do continuing bonds always help with adjustment to loss? *Bereavement Care* **21**(3): 41–2

Hancock S (2004) *The Two of Us: My Life with John Thaw.* Bloomsbury, London

Klass D, Silverman PR, Nickman SL (1996) *Continuing Bonds.* Taylor and Francis, Philadelphia

Kübler-Ross E (1969) *On Death and Dying.* Macmillan, New York

Lloyd-Williams M (ed) (2003) *Psychosocial Issues in Palliative Care.* OUP, Oxford

Oliviere D, Hargreaves R, Munroe B (1998) *Good Practices in Palliative Care: a Psychosocial Perspective.* Ashgate, Aldershot

Martin TL, Doka KJ (2000) *Men Don't Cry... Women Do.* Taylor and Francis, Philadelphia

Marwit SJ, Klass D (1995) Grief and the role of the inner representation of the deceased. *Omega* **30**: 283–98

NHS (2004) *Improving Supportive and Palliative Care for Adults with Cancer.* National Institute for Clinical Excellence (NICE), London

Parkes CM (1972) *Bereavement: Studies of Grief in Adult Life.* Penguin, Harmondsworth

Parkes CM (1986) *Bereavement: Studies of Grief in Adult Life.* 2nd edn. Routledge, London

Parkes CM (1996) *Bereavement: Studies of Grief in Adult Life.* 3rd edn. Routledge, London

Parkes CM, Weiss R (1983) *Recovery from Bereavement.* Basic Books, New York

Payne S, Horn S, Relf M (1999) *Loss and Bereavement.* Open University Press, Buckinghamshire

Payne S (2001) The role of volunteers in hospice bereavement support in New Zealand. *Palliat Med* **15**: 107–15

Relf M (1998) Involving volunteers in bereavement counselling. *Eur J Palliat Care* **5**: 61–5

Rossenblatt PC (1993) Grief: the social context of private feelings. In: Stroebe M, Stroebe W, Hanson RO (eds) *Handbook of Bereavement: Theory, Research and Intervention.* CUP, Cambridge

Shuchter SR, Zisook S (1993) The course of normal grief. In: Stroebe M, Stroebe W, Hanson RO (eds) *Handbook of Bereavement: Theory, Research and Intervention.* CUP, Cambridge

Stroebe M, Stroebe W, Hanson RO (eds) (1993) *Handbook of Bereavement: Theory, Research and Intervention.* CUP, Cambridge

Stroebe M (1997) From mourning and melancholia to bereavement and biography: an assessment of Walter's new model of grief. *Mortality* **2**(3): 255–62

Stroebe M (1998) New directions in bereavement research: exploration of gender differences. *Palliat Med* **12**: 5–12

Stroebe M, Schut H (1998) Culture and grief. *Bereavement Care* **17**(1): 7–11

Stroebe M, Schut H (1999) The dual process model of coping with bereavement: rationale and description. *Death Studies* **23**(3): 197–213

Walter T (1996) A new model of grief: bereavement and biography. *Mortality* **1**(1): 7–25

Walter T (1997) Letting go and keeping hold: a reply to Stroebe. *Mortality* **2**(3): 263–6

Worden JW (1982) *Grief Counselling and Grief Therapy.* Springer, New York

Worden JW (1991) *Grief Counselling and Grief Therapy.* 2nd edn. Springer, New York

Chapter 6

Interpersonal skills in palliative care social work

Nuala Cullen

Introduction

This chapter will look at the ways in which interpersonal communication occurs between professionals and service users within palliative care settings. The context of palliative care assumes a background of loss, change and adjustment in the lives of the client group. Theories of loss and change will be needed to provide a canvas for this chapter (see *Chapter 5*). People do not exist in isolation so, in one-to-one, couple, family or group interactions, there is always a wider context in the systems within which people, couples, families and groups function. Healthcare and, in particular, palliative care, as well as loss and change, become a key part of the system in which the person with a life-limiting illness and their family exists. The journey through healthcare is unique to the person and sometimes a whole new world is opened up to people who have little experience with healthcare settings, leading to further vulnerability in adjusting to the necessity of regular hospital visits and appointments.

The palliative care professional plays the role of facilitator in interpersonal communication with service users. People use interpersonal skills in daily interactions with each other in the usual context of life. It is expected that we might share our thoughts, worries and experiences with the people who are close to us in our lives. Less personal or intimate communication occurs with people we do not know very well or do not know at all. As professionals, we engage with people in a way that could, superficially, seem contrived or intrusive in asking that they share their personal thoughts, feelings, worries and concerns with a stranger. We are aware that there is often a great need for the person's experience to be heard. The task of the professional is to provide a safe environment in which a service user will feel comfortable in sharing their 'stuff'. This is what sets professional interpersonal communication apart from the interpersonal contact that people have in their daily lives, interacting with relatives and friends.

This chapter will explore ways in which professionals work towards relationship-building and skilled helping, leading to the provision of a listening, expressing and 'being' as well as a 'doing' service for people in palliative care settings. I will also look at the use of verbal and non-verbal communication. Listening skills and creative intervention will be examined against a backdrop of loss and systems theoretical approaches. I will do this by the use of case studies and will focus on practice issues.

Definitions

There are some all-encompassing or generic terms that can detract, at times, from the individuality of people if used uncritically. For the purposes of this chapter, I will use some of these terms, but in this section will explain what I mean by them. Terms such as 'the person', 'the carer' and the 'family' warrant careful definitions, which I ask the reader to bear in mind while reading.

By 'the person', I mean what the healthcare system describes as 'the patient'. It is important for the social worker to meet the 'person' first, and not to assume that the person is defined by their patient status. Often, in the healthcare journey that people experience, their status as patient is what defines them in the care world and becomes part of their identity, along with the illness with which they live. It is important for palliative care social workers to be sensitive to this fact and to work in a person-led way. Hence, the person might lead in talking about their illness if they choose, but will also have the freedom to lead to other areas of their current situation, their past and their future (Stroebe, 1995).

I use the term 'the carer' to refer to the individual who mainly looks after 'the person'. One must be aware that 'carers' may not refer to themselves as such, and indeed may not appreciate the label. 'Carers' might prefer to describe themselves as 'partner', 'husband', 'wife', 'sister', 'daughter', 'neighbour' and so on, with caring being a part of their role, rather than a role in itself. Some carers, however, may appreciate the acknowledgement of their caring role in being described as a 'carer'. Each 'carer' is unique, and their experience should be met without assumptions about their role and their motivation for engaging in it. It is also important to define 'care' widely — as being potentially practical, social, emotional and psychological (Nolan, Davies and Grant, 2000).

When I use the word 'family', I am aware of the diversity of families in contemporary society. Every family is different and, again, assumptions must be avoided. In this chapter, I use 'family' to mean the supportive network of people that surrounds 'the person'; I do not assume that this network will consist exclusively of blood relatives.

Loss and change

Palliative care takes place, in hospices, hospitals and home settings, for people for whom a journey through healthcare has occurred and for whom curative treatment is no longer an option (Twycross, 2003). Palliative care also exists for the support of family members of people in this position. For people to have reached a destination where palliative care is applicable, a series of losses and changes would usually be experienced. Reactions would occur to the progression of the illness in the minds and bodies of the people involved — both the person with the illness and the family system that surrounds them. These reactions may be very individual, but embody some similarities in how people adjust to loss and change (Bowlby, 1998).

Grief theory can be understood in the context of the series of losses that occur, from the diagnosis of an illness onwards to death and into bereavement (Oliviere *et al*, 1998). As the health journey proceeds, it may be helpful to understand grief work as a 'job' never done, and one that cannot be tidily managed; rather, each change brings a new wave of grief reactions, which create an altogether untidy picture of life with a life-threatening illness. Grief represents a loss or change in a person's significant attachments, and throws into question the meanings of their current and future relationships. For the carer and family, the future relationship with the person will be altered to be represented by memories, rather than the ongoing life one might have expected (Klass *et al*, 1996). Control is often what people in uncertain situations desire: they yearn for the familiar when they feel themselves lost. Some of the most familiar aspects of life are self, home and family. When a life-threatening illness invades, these are the very things that are threatened (Currer, 2000).

An understanding of the scale of the changes and losses that have already occurred in the journey is the foundation on which the social work relationship should be built with people with life-threatening illnesses and their families. The exploration of how someone has coped with a loss earlier in their journey may highlight some of the coping mechanisms available to them. It may reveal a vocabulary with which to work in order to access information about how the person is coping and feeling in the present, and what worries they might have about the future. Loss and change are ever-present factors in the lives of people with life-threatening illnesses and their families. The social worker explores with families, and with individuals within families, how the experience of loss and change is personal to them, and focuses the supportive role where it is needed. This might be in working with the family as a whole, or assessment might reveal a particular need for support with one or more individuals within the family.

Social work skills can help build relationships within which a person can feel supported in exploring their feelings about the losses they have experienced and the worries they may have. The case studies later in this chapter will shed further light on the role of the palliative care social worker. The social work role is as individual as the person or family with which social workers engage. Practical tasks may sometimes be involved, but the evolving relationship has lasting value. The relationship between the social worker and the person or people is central to the social work role. How does this relationship come to be?

Interpersonal skills

Interpersonal skills are the communication tools used in interactions between people. However, communication is enormously complex. It is difficult to understand the complexity of how we communicate within our own family networks. When we communicate with the people we know in our personal lives, we have a range of invisible rules and contracts about how we interact and what is 'normal' within each relationship. How is it, then, that as professionals, we enable the growth of relationships with one or more people within families with whom we have no personal relationship, but with whom we are likely to explore frightening areas of thought and feeling at a difficult time in the life of the person and family?

Again, in our personal lives, we are likely to be sensitive to the differences in our relationships with particular people and would pick up differences in a departure from 'normal' interactions. Our families and relationships within them might have different vocabularies to form a part of a distinct communication culture. Communication becomes a known or received system in how families interact with each other. As professionals, we cannot understand the intricate functioning of every family, but we can bear in mind that family functioning is complex, and that meeting families at times of stress is likely to exacerbate complexity and may lead to confusion (Thompson, 2002).

It is the basic acceptance of the uniqueness of individuals and families that is a foundation for how social workers use interpersonal skills to engage with people. Palliative care social work meets the person, carer and family without making assumptions of worth (Rogers, 1961). Before looking at how social workers might work with individuals and families, the core values of respect, a non-expert position and commitment to meeting people without assumption should be acknowledged as 'setting the scene' for how interpersonal communication might ensue.

The first contact one might have, as a professional in engaging with a person, carer or family, may not be in person at all. It might be that the person has been made aware of the social worker either by reading literature about the organisation or the service, or by being informed by a professional from another discipline that a social worker may contact them. It is important to be aware of the potential expectations someone might have about meeting the social worker, and to be sensitive to the need to explain the relationship, clearing up any misunderstandings that might arise. There might be a need to check out a person's thoughts about seeing a social worker and what they think it will mean to them. Exploring their expectations and perceptions will indicate to the person, carer or family that they have some say in the relationship and the support that will be offered.

For example, a person might respond to a question about what expectations they have about the social work role by saying that they would expect their benefits to be sorted out. The social worker might reply that this could indeed be part of the role, but that, just as everyone's social circumstances are different, the social work role can be as individual as the person. This means that the role can address financial and practical issues, but can also provide emotional support and an opportunity to explore worries, concerns, thoughts and feelings with individuals and families.

Alternatively, the space and time that the social worker shares with the individual need not be anything more than that — shared space and time. The message the social worker gives to the person, the carer and the family is that every experience is valid and that the experience of life-threatening or life-limiting illness is one that touches the entire family network, sometimes changing family roles in a context of ongoing loss (Sheldon, 1997). The messages that the person, carer and family should hear loud and clear from the social worker at the outset of any interpersonal professional relationship are that they and their experience are being respected and valued. When conflict exists within families, this remains the outset need in forming relationships. These are the fundamental introductory factors that set the scene for any relationship that follows. As the interpersonal relationship grows, appropriate challenging will be enabled in a safe environment, but the relationship should be based on respect and value.

Interpersonal skills in this context require an ability to listen and to hear the person, carer and family. 'Listen' and 'hear' are, again, apparently simple words that have complex meanings in our interactions with people, carers and families. The interpersonal skills of the professional may also help a family by creating a space in which listening and hearing between family members can take place (see *Case study 3*). We are not merely listening to the words that people are saying: there is also a need to consider the actions and interactions of people; to hear what is not being said and to ask sensitively the right questions in response (Rowe, 1996). Some of the complexities of the listening role include:

- silence
- resistance
- difference
- body language
- explanation.

Silence

Silence is an interesting experience to share. In our busy, must-do world, silence might seem wasteful, as time spent in interacting with others is often considered to be purposeful and outcome-led. One wonders, however, what happens behind the silence as it is being shared. Indeed, it is important to acknowledge that a process occurs when a silence is shared. As a social worker visiting a service user, there is an expectation of purpose, so that when silence is shared, it becomes a skill to feel comfortable with it. Silence should be valued, but how can this be listening?

In silence, what one is listening to is the person communicating a need not to talk; a need to think whilst being witnessed and valued in safety; or a need not to share thoughts. It might be that one could revisit, and discuss with the service user at a later time, what processes he or she was experiencing during the silence, or to find out whether it was a valuable time. Alternatively, maybe it does not need to be defined and can just be time shared together that does not need to be explained? One might be sensitive to what is not being said as a communication from somebody. It might be that a significant fact about health status or family relationships is clear, but that the subject is avoided. This might be communicating that the person is not ready to discuss the subject, or that you are not the person they want to discuss it with. Again, one must respect the person's truth as they display it.

Resistance

Resistance is a familiar experience in social work practice. We must ask, however — what is being communicated with resistance and how is resistance being displayed? Challenging behaviour and cancelled or unattended visits are some ways in which service users might resist social-work contact. We must also ask — what is the source of resistant behaviours? Is it perhaps fear of what will be discussed or expected, or confusion over what social work is all about? In practice, one must be aware of less evident strategies of resistance, such as a person talking so much that the social worker cannot interact; answering a question that has not being asked; or avoiding one that has. It is vital to remember that resistance is communicating something, and this might be something that could be explored when (or if) the time is right for the person (Parker, 2003). It may also mean, simply, that the service user does not wish to work with you. This is something of which social workers must also be mindful.

Difference

Difference is communication. Social workers should be sensitive to differences from 'the norm' in what a person is saying or doing, or in how they are interacting with others. Crucially, the communication consists in the difference that has occurred. One can notice the difference as a difference in itself, and use it as a reflection to ask the person what they think it might mean. In *Case study 2*, I will examine how the difference in Sean's eating patterns helped us explore his feelings.

Body language

Body language is a powerful means of communication both in an individual's interactions with us as social workers and in their interactions with other people. Eye-contact, how the body is positioned, and hand and body movements, for example, might reveal pain, anger and anxiety, as well as comfort and relaxation. Professionals should be aware of what their own bodies are communicating. Our self-awareness in this, as in all interpersonal communications, is key to successful relationship-building with the person, carer and family.

Explanation

The words and vocabulary that people use open doors for communication. There might be a need to define what is meant by particular words — for example, when metaphors are used. Someone might say that they are 'lost'. What does this mean to them? When were they not 'lost'? Someone might respond to 'How are you?' by saying 'Fine'. What does 'Fine' mean to them? What is it like when they are not 'Fine'? The meaning of words can be used as a gentle way of challenging and widening the scope of the exchange with the person.

Interpersonal skills are required in creatively guiding our interactions with people and being sensitive to where people will go in their communications, and when they want to go no further. The facilitation of relationship-building needs to be skilfull. People should be assured that they are being heard and listened to. It might be that the professional would reflect, summarise or notice aloud what they have heard or seen, sending the message that the speaker has been listened to, respected and valued (Egan, 1998). It is important to probe appropriately in the search for understanding the person's experience or story, and also to be honest about not having understood and needing help where necessary in order to understand more fully.

The use of interpersonal skills in palliative care social work is key to the unique relationships social workers have with this client group. The fundamentals of respect and value are the base upon which relationship-building with the person, the carer and the family takes place in this setting. Allowing the 'being' as well as 'doing' role gives permission for the relationship itself to be valuable without assumptions about what will be achieved. However, as we shall see, communication does not just take place between individuals, but also between wider groups of people. The larger systems involved in the palliative care process are complex and important.

Systems theory

Families can be viewed as systems, understanding the impact of life-threatening illness and bereavement on all members of the family. Simplistically, one could understand life-threatening illness as something that happens to the person with the illness, and bereavement as something experienced by the carer and family. There could exist a hierarchy of importance, depending on the relationship with the deceased, so that a spouse would be the 'most' bereaved and an adult sibling 'less' bereaved.

However, such ideas fail to appreciate the complexity of families. If one views a family as a system, one acknowledges that each person is a component within the system with a unique part to play. In functioning, the experience of one component impacts on others within the system. Components cannot function in isolation. When changes occur to one part of the system, the system adjusts to the change. If one understands families in this way, it is clear that when a life-threatening illness is experienced by one person in the family, it becomes part of the system and impacts on the whole (Payne, 2005).

The impact of a life-threatening illness on a family system is clearly shown in *Case study 1*. If grief is the response to loss, and loss occurs in life with a life-threatening illness, then clearly the family for whom life-threatening illness is an issue begins to grieve, including the person who is physically experiencing the illness. Each member of the family has a different perception and experience of current and future losses. The person experiencing the illness faces progressive physical losses and, ultimately, the loss of life at an uncertain time. This person may grieve for self and family at a very vulnerable and medically busy time. The experience of the carer may be the expectation of engaging in roles that are unfamiliar, while also living with the worry about the future beyond the death of the person with the illness. Often, the busy caring role leaves little space for self, and carers can become physically and emotionally exhausted in adjusting to a life-threatening illness in the system. They may get smothered in their new identity as they engage in the caring role and lose sight of who they perceive themselves to be in the confusion of a grieving system.

The impact of life-threatening illness on a family system can be far-reaching. Understanding the experience from a systems perspective gives the professional a wide view of the adjusting family who are being affected by a shared experience in an individual way. By gaining an understanding of how the family system works, social workers are in a position to empower the family to explore the dynamics with which they live and interact, and to consider how other family members are being affected by the illness. The case studies illustrate this point further.

Case study 1: Laura

Laura is a forty-four year-old mother of two children, aged ten and twenty-one years. She was diagnosed with throat cancer eight months ago and had surgery, which removed her voice box. She now talks, with difficulty and discomfort, through her 'tracheotomy'. When approached by the social worker, she said that she was fine, though a bit fed up about the loss of her voice, and indicated that she wanted further contact. She has difficulties with reading and writing.

In this case, Laura was verbally communicating that she would like to have further contact after our introductory meeting. No agenda was identified at this point, but a second visit was arranged. I noted with Laura her difficulty in talking and the discomfort she was experiencing, and asked whether she would like to work with something visual when we met; Laura agreed.

On the second visit, we looked at Laura's positioning within her family network, using a genogram and representing family members by the use of magazine cut-outs. (A genogram is an informative family tree, which visually represents the family network — see Parker and Bradley, 2003.) Laura identified a symbol from a magazine that represented to her a family member, and this was stuck to a large piece of paper to construct the genogram. Laura found this exercise fun and valued having a visual representation of her family and her roles and positioning within it.

We decided to continue to use this medium to create a collage of feeling for Laura, around the genogram, that represented her experience with her illness and its impact on her relationships with her children. Laura tapped into the experience of others within the family and developed an understanding of her illness having a wider impact on other members of the family. Over a period of weeks, Laura was able to explore, process, acknowledge and validate some of her feelings and was also pleased with having produced a piece of work — a colourful collage — that was very meaningful to her, that was private and abstract in content, and that was her individual representation of her experience in the family context.

This medium was suitable to Laura due to a need to work visually because of her discomfort with talking, and her difficulties with reading and writing. Essentially, this was a representation of a family system in transition. Laura's illness had entered the family system and began to affect emotionally and pyschologically Laura and her family, both as individuals and as 'parts' of a system. Family roles were adjusting to the changing situation; these adjustments felt scary and unstable for family members.

Genograms are a powerful means with which to explore family dynamics and and to create a visual representation of each family member's place. Genograms can be used as information-gathering tools, but are very useful in one-to-one and family work. Some other ways of looking visually at relationships within families include ecomaps (which show relationships and their strengths) and the use of Russian dolls. These also embody family systems theory and can establish family dynamics in a non-threatening way. Issues such as power dynamics within families and levels of attachment within relationships can be explored by this approach. Systems theory enables an acknowledgement of the experience of each individual involved in the immediate system. In a palliative care context, as discussed earlier, loss and change play a role in the family system. The social work role is enriched by the understanding of the individual, contextualised by their unique family system and the dynamics within it.

Case study 2: Sean

Sean is a sixty-five year-old man who is the husband of a day patient at the local hospice. Sean has health problems too and has recovered from cancer in the past. He is also diabetic. On first assessment with the social worker, Sean's coping mechanisms were explored. Sean said that he tries to keep himself busy, but finds late evenings difficult when it is quiet and his thoughts 'sneak up on him'. He said that he tends to eat more biscuits than he should at these quiet times and he worries about the effects of this. He said that he is aware that he is 'bottling things up', and that he tries to avoid thinking too much by keeping busy and active. He asked for further contact and the social worker made a further appointment.

On second meeting, I shared with Sean my reflections on our first conversations. There were two things that had been 'bubbling in my head': the first was that Sean was neglecting his own health and making himself vulnerable (especially in light of his diabetes) by eating biscuits; the second was that, when he had said that he was 'bottling things up', what did he think was in the bottle, where did he think the bottle was, and did he have any ideas about how he would empty the bottle if it got too full?

I wondered, along with Sean, whether there were any connections between these two things, reflecting that Sean had said that he tried to keep himself distracted from the 'bottled-up' feelings and that distractions were more difficult to find in the evenings when he was alone. I wondered whether the eating of the biscuits was serving as another distraction from the thoughts that were 'sneaking up'. Sean commented that he found this hypothesis interesting and agreed for us to explore, so to speak, what was in his bottle. I suggested that we draw a bottle and write in it what it contained. Sean asked that I do the drawing and writing and that he would guide me in what the bottle contained. Sean said that he felt the bottle was inside him and was very big, even though he did not want to give it attention.

Sean revealed the loss of a significant relationship, as well as other losses that 'filled' a large part of the bottle. There was a strong feeling of 'What else can go wrong?' in the bottle. Some feelings that were attached to these included worry, fear, disbelief, numbness, a need to escape and the question 'Why?' We explored what it felt like for Sean to look at what was in the bottle, and Sean said that looking at it helped to empty it a little. I asked him whether there might be anyone in his support network that could help him empty it more regularly; he did not feel there was anyone. I said I would be willing temporarily to fill that role and arranged further sessions where we would look at the bottle but also consider other ways for Sean to empty it. He agreed to monitor his intake of biscuits by making a note of the quantity and time of eating, and to pay attention to his thoughts and feelings at the times when he reached for the biscuit tin. This encouraged jim to listen to his own behaviour and develop an understanding of this behaviour.

The exploration, validation and normalisation of thoughts and feelings are part of the domain of the social worker in palliative care settings. People often carry thoughts in their heads that they do not want to have or even acknowledge. As social workers, we do not always need to know what these are for the people with whom we work. But we might remember that unwanted thoughts and feelings are often an aspect of life for people in their position, and that though they may or may not be having them, such thoughts and feelings are normal and valid. This witnessing and normalisation of thoughts and feelings can be done whether or not the person chooses to share them verbally.

Often, people will say, in the context of living with difficulty, that they just 'get through one day at a time'. The 'how' is the indicator of coping skills: how do they get through it one day at a time? Is it possible not to think about the past and the future in the context of a difficult 'now'? The exploration of a person's eating and sleeping patterns can reveal differences in habit and lifestyle that speak volumes for a person in Sean's position. Unwanted thoughts and feelings can do their 'sneaking up' around sleeping routines, and really have an impact even when someone is trying to deny them. The observation of difference in how a person may be functioning in their routines, and an exploration of what impact the difference might be having, are example of how difference can be a way of communicating. This is akin to Beck's identification of automatic negative thoughts (Beck, 1976): the social work role is to ensure that alternative and more constructive thought-patterns are identified.

The use of words and language is shown in Sean's case by using his metaphor 'bottling up'. By checking out meaning and bringing his metaphor to life, a space was created in which Sean started to explore the very things he said he kept so busy to avoid and found the experience helpful. In this narrative approach, the social worker adopts a non-expert position in which meaning is determined by the person, and the person leads the way.

Case study 3: The Wilson family

Mr Wilson died at home two weeks ago after a long and increasingly deteriorating illness. Mrs Wilson and her three teenage daughters are now in early bereavement. Mrs Wilson has contacted the hospice Family Support Team requesting a home visit to the family. Mrs Wilson has explained that she feels that family members are finding it difficult to talk about their experiences and suspects that her daughters are 'putting on a brave face', as she is.

I visited the Wilson family at home, with a plan to undertake a family session around feelings and support networks. I thought I might uncover what feelings were around for family members and explore what was helping family members cope (looking at therapeutic and distractive elements of coping). I suggested that we do this as a paper, as well as a verbal exercise. I shared my plan with the family and asked whether they would like to pursue my plan; they agreed.

I asked each family member to write their names on a piece of paper. I then asked them to place these in a circle, ensuring that there was some available space in the centre. I provided many smaller pieces of paper. I invited family members to bring to mind one or more other members of the family in the session. I invited them to consider for a few moments what feelings might have been around for them in recent weeks. I asked that they write what they would guess to be the feelings of others, with one feeling per piece of paper. (They were not asked to identify who they were thinking of). I then asked for people to put the feelings into the centre of the circle. The family studied these for a while, remarking on how many similarities there were, in that there were several 'angers', 'guilts' and 'sadnesses', among others.

I then provided more pieces of paper and invited family members to think about what had helped them to cope or feel supported in the previous weeks. I asked them to think about the people in their lives, and also the things that they do. I asked them to think about who and what helps them to think about the difficult issues, and who and what helps distract them (bearing in mind that this could all be embodied in one person or activity). I asked that this 'blue circle' — the paper was blue — be placed as an outer circle as a representation of the family's support network. Visually, this represented the feelings in the centre directly affecting the family circle, who were being supported by the 'blue circle'. I explored with the family how the feelings might change, and also how the blue circle might change, but stressed that it was important to be aware that they are there. *Figure 6.1* shows this visual way of working.

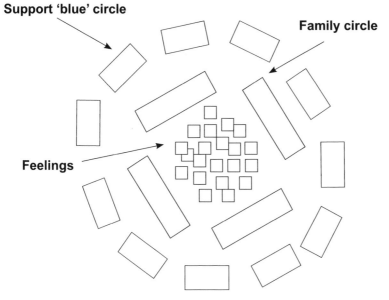

Figure 6.1: Visual representation of feelings in the Wilson family (*Case study 3*)

Initial information in this case study revealed that Mrs Wilson felt worried that people might have difficulty talking about their experience. This assessment was useful in planning the session, in that taking the pressure off talking and doing a paper exercise instead may have felt more comfortable. Also, by being invited to consider others' feelings rather than their own, there were elements of distancing and freeing of indviduals from the experience of owning their feelings. Rather, the session revealed the feelings that were currently alive in the family system, and acknowledged them in a non-threatening way. Feelings were normalised, validated and noticed as common to the experience of others in the system. Mr Wilson was still a very big part of this system and the impact of his absence and the changes this necessitated for family members were what was being represented. Again, this family found it helpful to have something visual and external, and the exercise opened up a space in which individuals began to share verbally their thoughts and feelings with each other.

The creation by the family of their 'blue circle' helped them identify the ways in which they were being supported. Acknowledging both distractive and therapeutic support and coping mechanisms allows a rounded view of coping, so that people can look internally (into themselves) as well as externally (into other people) to explore all the things that help.

Conclusion

This chapter has looked at ways in which effective interpersonal skills in palliative care social work maximise the value of the relationship with the person, the carer and the family. Three case studies have shown some ways in which creative interpersonal skills can provide a basis for effective working relationships. Key themes in this chapter have been communication and systems thinking in relation to people with life-threatening illnesses, carers and families. Interpersonal skills and relationships are grounded in communication and communication is grounded in the listening role. This chapter has highlighted the importance of acknowledging the complexities of the listening role. Such complexities were discussed, including the importance of listening to behaviour and also to silence, resistance, difference, body language and explanation (or the meanings people give to the vocabulary they use).

The case studies showed the importance of being individual in the use of interpersonal skills. The Wilson family, in *Case study 3*, illustrated how a bereaved family were enabled to create a space within which they could communicate with each other in a way that had been avoided. They were encouraged to tap into their listening skills by naming the feelings that they thought other members of the family were having. An open discussion about feelings had not occurred, but the family accurately assessed the feelings of other members and began a valuable discussion about the impact of the illness and death of Mr Wilson. Through the exploration of the meaning of words, Sean, in *Case study 2*, developed his 'bottling up' metaphor to become a useful tool with which his feelings were explored. Creative communication with Laura, in *Case study 1*, in doing something visual rather than having the pressure of talking, enabled the social work relationship to grow.

The second key theme of this chapter has been the use of systems thinking in looking at illness and death in families. The importance of being individual in the use of interpersonal skills remains, but systems theory takes this a step further to place the individual in their unique context with the family network around them and the loss and change they experience. This enables the social worker and family to develop an understanding of the impact of life-threatening illness on the whole family network, and respond to this in an individual way. Systems theory is shown by the case studies, particularly that of Laura. Through genogram work, she was able to develop some understanding of her own experience, but was also able to acknowledge the impact her illness may have been having on her children. She felt that this helped her to understand some of the behaviour the children had been exhibiting. Likewise, in the Wilson family, the family system was acknowledged for the feelings inside it and the support network, 'the blue circle', around it.

It is clear that interpersonal skills are as complex as the individuals who use them. Given that they are part of everyday communication with people, it may be tempting to undervalue the role of interpersonal skills in a professional context. However, the ability to create a space within which a person is listened to and valued in a non-judgemental way is a core aspect of palliative care social work, and is fundamental to effective and ethical practice.

References

Beck A (1976) *Cognitive Therapy and the Emotional Disorders.* International University Press, New York

Bowlby J (1998) *Attachment and Loss: Attachment.* Pimlico edn. Pimlico, London

Currer C (2000) *Responding to Grief: Dying, Bereavement and Social Care.* Palgrave, Basingstoke

Egan G (1998) *The Skilled Helper.* 6th edn. Brooks/Cole, London

Nolan M, Davies S, Grant G (eds) (2000) *Working with Older People and their Families: Key Issues in Policy and Practice.* Open University Press, Buckinghamshire

Klass D, Silverman PR, Nickman SL (1996) *Continuing Bonds: New Understandings of Grief.* Taylor & Francis, London

Oliviere D, Hargreaves R, Monroe B (1998) *Good Practices in Palliative Care: a Psychosocial Perspective.* Ashgate/Arena, Aldershot

Parker J (2003) Positive communication with people who have dementia. In: Adams T, Manthorpe J (eds) *Dementia Care.* Arnold, London

Parker J, Bradley G (2003) *Social Work Practice: Assessment, Planning, Intervention and Review.* Learning Matters, Exeter

Payne M (2005) *Modern Social Work Theory.* 3rd edn. Palgrave, Basingstoke

Rogers C (1961) *On Becoming a Person: a Therapist's View of Psychotherapy.* Constable, London

Rowe D (1996) *Depression: the Way Out of Your Prison.* Routledge, London

Sheldon F (1997) *Psychosocial Palliative Care: Good Practices in the Care of the Dying and Bereaved.* Nelson Thornes, Cheltenham

Stroebe W, Stroebe MS (1995) *Social Psychology and Health.* Open University Press, Buckinghamshire

Thompson N (ed) (2002) *Loss and Grief: a Guide to Human Services Practitioners.* Palgrave, Basingstoke

Twycross R (2003) *Introducing Palliative Care.* 4th edn. Radcliffe, Oxford

Chapter 7

Dramatherapy in palliative care

Andy Bird

*Our relationships with our parents and partners, friends and children,
make us die numerous little deaths and equally make us live through
numerous resurrections long before we encounter death itself.*

(Gersie, 1991: 28)

Introduction

In this chapter, I will draw on my knowledge and experience to illustrate the
essential themes of 'ending' while working with terminally ill people in a
hospice in the north of England. (I use the words 'end' or 'ending' to refer to
drawing a piece of work to a close; and also in a more popular sense to denote
a significant change or break in a relationship, which may, at times, be death.) I
will integrate my personal reflections and experience with acquired wisdom of
what promotes a good ending. I will explore how an awareness of an approaching
ending prepares us better to manage and cope with it. I will develop the notions
of honesty and authenticity as integral to healthy relationships and central to a
good ending, so that a new journey can begin.

Life is unpredictable, so planning for unexpected events is not always
possible. We cannot always forsee the redundancy, loss of status, sudden death
and separation that an ending may bring. Unexpected loss does not permit the
psychological preparation needed to make a complete and necessary goodbye
— a goodbye that expresses our feelings towards someone (or something)
with whom we have developed a significant bond. We can be left unable to
integrate the shocking news, in denial, and unprepared to make a good ending.
Consequently, we may have unfinished business, carrying unacknowledged
feelings and thoughts in our conscious and unconscious mind, which hold us
back and prevent us living in the present. Being able to foresee or plan an ending
could be considered an honour, therefore, because it offers an opportunity to
let go of the past and move on. For Renee Emunah (1996: 38), a 'carefully
designed process of closure' can help 'integrate the past, but creates a sense of
opening to the future'.

The importance of good endings

A carefully prepared ending is an opportunity to process the five phases of loss famously formulated by Elisabeth Kübler-Ross (1970) in her work with terminally ill people: denial, anger, bargaining, depression and acceptance of one's fate. These phases enable one to acclimatise to the loss, which is part of the grief process. Parkes (1996: 167) writes that '"grief work" is "making real" the fact of loss'. A good end, therefore, enables a person to adjust to the facts of separation and the need to find sense and meaning in what has happened.

'Finding meaning' is essential in grief work, since it facilitates the process of integrating the loss into daily life and adapting to living without the significant person. No two people grieve alike: finding meaning in loss is unique to every individual and intensifies our differences. A good ending legislates for an individual process of grief, allowing for a unique engagement and expression of loss.

Graham

I worked with an adolescent boy, Graham, to whom I offered ten sessions of therapeutic work regarding the death of his mother. As we neared the end of our therapeutic work, he disengaged and stopped attending. After a telephone conversation, we agreed that I could visit him in his own home, where he felt it was possible to close the work in a way that was appropriate and unique to him. He decided on lighting two candles that symbolically represented to him our relationship. In semi-darkness and in silence, we observed the lit candles, while Graham, with clasped hands, appeared to be praying quietly.

At the time to part, we blew out the candles to signify the end. Throughout, I was conscious that the ritual may also have symbolically represented a 'closure' with his mother that he may have been unable to make previously. The ritual might have enabled him to process the separation in the here and now, with myself as therapist potentially representing his mother. The closing ritual he devised offered the distance and safety he needed to make a good ending that had meaning for her. He was able to cope with our separation by choosing to make a more indirect and symbolic goodbye that offered the possibility to close other relationships he had been unable to close. In this way, Graham maintained some control over potentially overwhelming feelings, making his own sense of ending, regardless of what it meant to me. The importance of control in endings is explored in Wilson, Kendrick and Ryan (1992: 130) who recognise the importance of the young person having a choice over the ending, rather then being told by the therapist how to end.

Sogyal Rinpoche, a Tibetan Buddhist monk, emphasises a peaceful death to help the dead person on their new journey, using a purification ritual so that any ill feeling or violence at the time of the death will not have karmic consequences for a rebirth (Rinpoche, 1992: 305). I think this also illustrates the importance of good ending, so that past ill feelings are not carried unresolved into new relationships. The importance of peace chimes with Kübler-Ross's 'acceptance phase', where the dying patient is given enough time to 'express feelings about their fate' and mourn 'impending losses' (Kübler-Ross, 1970: 99).

However, in my hospice work, some patients were regarded as 'difficult', because of their hostility or anger, which resulted in them being ignored or even avoided by staff. Consequently, these patients became isolated and the gulf between the living and the dying was widened.

The reverse should have been the case. It is important that we 'learn to listen to our patients and at times even to accept some irrational anger, knowing that the relief in expressing it will help them toward a better acceptance of the final hours' (Kübler-Ross, 1970: 48). Endings can be uncomfortable for the therapist and client alike, but recognising that they trigger painful and existential issues means we can be more empathetic to our clients' predicament and more attentive to what might appear to be irrational anger.

Graham expressed a lot of anger towards me as the ending of our work approached, but I felt I made ending tolerable for him because I was able to hold his feelings and help him manage what could have been a potentially overwhelming experience.

Good endings

Good endings allow children and adults to share their feelings without fear of upsetting anyone; consequently, they need not face the unknown while anxious and alone. Irvin Yalom (1985: 23), in his work with cancer patients, writes: 'what the patient needs is contact, to be able to voice concerns openly, to be reminded that he or she is not only "apart from" but also "a part of"'. In my hospice work, I have been moved by the warmth, honesty and openness in families — to such an extent that being in their presence cut through the superficiality of life, creating good conditions to die.

On the other hand, I have seen how families can create a divide from the patient because they do not wish them to know they are dying or have cancer, creating isolation and loneliness and making a good ending difficult. However, it is important to respect how people cope with endings, whether it appears unhealthy or not, and nobody has any right to undermine a person's need to protect themselves. A good ending recognises that different people cope with grief and endings in a multitude of ways, some approaches appearing more conducive then others. We have to remember that any coping strategy is an attempt to:

> *succeed in mastering the problem, and may at times become distorted or pathological,* [but this] *does not detract from its proper function, which is presumably the restoration of a control by distancing an individual from a situation that threatens to become overwhelming.*
>
> (Parkes, 1996: 73).

However, as a facilitator of endings, I feel it's important to take a degree of risk so that the best possible ending can be achieved. Graham's simple candle ritual was his way of closing a relationship in the present and possibly in the past. We should also remember that some clients are unable even to attend the final session — unable to confront the end in any overt way.

Children who have not been allowed to make an appropriate ending with a loved one who has died may prove problematic for making and maintaining other significant relationships because of unresolved closure. According to Jewett (1984: 13), children are 'liable to sustain additional damage to their basic sense of trust and security'. This could be illustrated with Graham, who, on his mother's death, had a problematic and volatile relationship with his father. At the end of the closing ritual, he was able to acknowledge to his father the anger he felt at being deprived of the opportunity to view his dead mother. He was not given an appropriate opportunity to confront his grief and, consequently, directed his anger towards his father, who had denied him closure. A safe ending and separation is important, although it is crucial that the child or young person is allowed to dictate what their idea of 'safety' is.

Looking after yourself in endings

The therapist, in my experience, is as prone as the patient to the denial of painful feelings when working with endings. For the therapist to be honest and authentic about his or her sadness helps facilitate and sanction the patient's feelings about loss, separation and death. As Mackay (1996: 173) writes: 'I am not merely the therapist; they are not merely patients: we are people who have travelled together'. In my personal experience of positive endings, they promote a real relationship with the patient, where a deeper level of communication becomes possible, reinforcing the bond and connection. A good ending has something of Clarkson's (1995: 191) 'transpersonal' psychotherapy about it — which is 'beyond rationality, facts and theories', entering the realm of 'the spiritual, the metaphysical, the mystical', making a good ending unique, intimate and special.

I have found that endings are often full of inexplicable tendencies and tensions, some of which can be traced back to earlier experiences of endings, which affect the present.

Personally, my earliest experience of loss was the death of my uncle. My mother protected me from the knowledge and impact of his death by telling me he was ill. I was aware of my own tendency and desire to 'rescue' patients when ending the 'therapeutic relationship' from what I imagined would be an overwhelming feeling of loss. However, being aware of how my previous experiences of loss might affect me and the client, I was able to facilitate the client's grieving process with an awareness of my own potential issues, thereby reducing the likelihood of my own process interfering. In this way, I was able to concentrate on the client's process and support him or her more effectively. Disclosing some of my sadness about separation to Graham offered him the opportunity to acknowledge his feelings, thereby enabling him to learn healthy grieving without resorting to 'stiff upper lip' attitudes adopted by some adults, and therefore recognising 'normal' feelings (Parkes, 1996: 145). In this way, it was an honour to offer Graham an ending that was open and honest, where he could develop his own response to loss and not worry about 'holding himself together'.

A good ending requires the therapist not to mask uncomfortable feelings with a 'potential lie or myth' (Yalom, 1980) and allowing individuals their own responses to loss. This helps with the development of the necessary skills and resources needed to master the conflicting emotions in their unique grief, as no two people grieve alike. Respecting each individual experience of endings is paramount and brings to mind a comment by a tutor, working with people living with HIV and AIDS, who said: 'if you can't be honest with the dying, who can you be honest with?'. I consider a good ending a time for being honest because ending affords moments for authentic living.

Drama and play — the search for meaning

The following case example illustrates a patient's search for meaning by means of a process that used small objects in a non-directive and client-centred manner. The process involved creating miniature staged scenes that helped the client tell his or her story in symbolic form. Although the process gave the patient the opportunity to explore what they perceived as most pressing, I offered the patient a basic structure to help contain feelings safely.

Offering the patient a client-centred approach can be less threatening because they are able to sustain the necessary defence mechanisms required to support the exploration on their own terms, thereby reducing anxiety. Confronting death produces anxiety because it represents the unknown. Fransella and Dalton (2000: 40) write: 'anxiety is thus an inevitable companion of change.

For whenever we put ourselves into a new situation, we must be faced with new events which we are likely to have difficulty construing'. Therefore, any potential exploration of death needs to be client-centred, taking the lead from the client and responding to their prompts.

The patient is given a sheet of A4 paper, then asked to choose from a selection of everyday objects — small animals, stones and figures — that represent their feelings, and locating them on the paper. The patient then explains what each object represents to them and why they chose it. Playing with objects in this manner helps the client to explore their feelings in a playful and indirect way. Winnicott (1971: 41) writes: 'it is play that is universal, and that belongs to health. Playing facilitates growth, and therefore health'. Just as children play to make discoveries of their world, so adults play to facilitate exploration. The objects act as a metaphor, distancing the client from their direct experience and minimising the potentially overwhelming feelings that often surround death. The client is thus able to project and attribute any difficult issues or emotions on to the object, protecting himself or herself in the meantime. Duggan and Grainger (1997: 23) write: 'metaphor provides us with a way of expressing the otherwise inexpressible'.

It becomes easier for the patient to project his or her burden onto, for example, a heavy stone and talk about how heavy the stone is in the hand than to talk directly about the burden the patient carries in day-to-day living. Being able to pick up the stone in the hand, put it down, feel it and describe it makes it tangible and visible. This leads to a sense of mastery and control over the burden or issue because it can be seen, touched and played with; consequently, the issues can be articulated and explored more readily. Gersie (1991: 235) writes, 'the act of making something also furthers our sense of mastery, and paradoxically helps us to consent to "newness"'. Having a feeling of mastery leads to a sense of control over one's life, when potentially there is little control over the surmounting changes and losses associated with living with a terminal illness. Using objects as metaphors enables clients to find meaning about life and death safely, while empowering them with the ability to 'express the inexpressible'.

Maureen

Maureen was an in-care patient in a hospice. She seemed depressed and withdrawn. Although she was physically mobile, she chose to spend most of her time in bed. Maureen came to my attention because of her imminent discharge home and her unhappiness about this decision. But she returned home nevertheless, where she lived on her own, supported appropriately by friends and family. It was from home that my work with Maureen began, offering her a contract of four sessions using the miniature-stages approach.

The first session

In the first session, Maureen was receptive and reflective, choosing objects to represent her present feelings. Objects on the paper represented home, friends, security and her late husband. The theme of the scene seemed to be loss, which was reinforced by a small animal used to represent Maureen's dog, for which she could no longer care. Maureen's exploration and discussion centred around the recent loss of her dog, which represented a very close friend. One object was placed outside the paper's edge that seemed to cause some distress to Maureen. She stressed that the object represented a stepdaughter who had caused her a lot of upset, and she was therefore placed at the periphery of the paper. Maureen entitled the scene 'friendship'.

It seemed to make some sense that the stepdaughter who was upsetting Maureen should not be part of the picture, but it did illustrate the conflicts in the family system. Maureen was beginning to find some meaning in the scene from her everyday life. Seeing her world represented on paper helped her bring clarity and understanding to her life, recognising the source of some of her pain, and possible depression. Being able physically to pick up and locate some of the pain symbolically though the objects gave her a sense of being able to manage her pain and control it more effectively. Through the use of dramatic metaphor, Maureen was able to express feelings that may have proved too difficult to express directly. Jennings (1997: 238) writes: 'Through the dramatic enactment, people may express thoughts and feelings that cannot be expressed in direct verbal ways'.

The second session

In the second session, Maureen developed a story using the objects. However, she felt unable to fictionalise a story. The story she did create was similar to past ones about her dog with some variations, but a new theme emerged around loss.

Her story was about the ending of her relationship with her dog. Maureen was very upset and was working through her loss at her own pace and in her own way, with appropriate guidance and support from me as her therapist. Although Maureen was able to make connections between her real-life experiences and the objects, I was particularly interested in her concerns about fictionalising a story. I felt Maureen was responding well and so I wanted to encourage her to work more with metaphor and fiction in her work, because I felt the safety of fiction or metaphor would help her explore her feelings better. I sensed from her work at the end of the session that Maureen wanted to approach her feelings about her own impending end. Although it was only a hunch, and I had no concrete evidence, I wanted her to have every opportunity to be able to take the exploration wherever she wanted. By making simple observations, I was able to keep the possibilities alive so Maureen could respond and direct her work in any chosen direction.

The third session

Still maintaining client choice and a person-centred approach in the third session, I developed a new angle to work with Maureen. Before she used the objects, I did some relaxation and guided imagery work, where I encouraged Maureen to visualise a stage with a play on it. My intention was to help her relax sufficiently so that she could use more of her senses and access her imaginative and creative selves, as I believed these would help her problem-solving abilities. After the visualisation, I asked Maureen to pick one moment in the play and, using the objects, represent the props, staging and characters that featured. The scene was in Malta, outside a church. Maureen portrayed a path that led to a cross where Jesus Christ hung. To the side of the path was Mary, the mother of Christ, with whom Maureen identified strongly. To emphasise the fictional nature of the story, and thereby guard Maureen's 'emotional safety', I encouraged her to address the character as Mary, not as herself, as she had been inclined to do.

Animals surrounded the scene with which Maureen had made an important connection. Generally, the scene was crowded; the paper representing the stage was almost full with objects. The picture had relevance for Maureen, but she herself wasn't entirely sure what it meant. Object by object, Maureen explored the part and role each played in the play. The theme of friendship was still present, but the context of the scene had changed, and the theme of death was becoming more prominent. The object Maureen had chosen for the path to the church seemed to resemble a coffin, but this was only my perception: to Maureen it was a path. It was important not to challenge Maureen's story, as this could obscure its meaning for her. Sometimes, a therapist can feel a strong temptation to interrupt a patient's story to find out a meaning that, in reality, may have little or no benefit for the patient. By resisting this temptation, I was able to uphold a client-centred approach.

Maureen was animated and energised as she talked about the scene, expressing amazement at some discoveries and uncertainty and curiousity about others. Maureen was given the opportunity to make any changes she wanted to make to the scene, but felt that the scene was complete.

She dismantled the scene carefully, returning the objects to the box until she was left with a blank piece of paper again. When summing up the scene, I asked Maureen to give the scene a caption. She entitled it, 'Half ending story'. I had felt that Maureen was beginning to explore her own death, but the caption suggested that had not yet finished her exploration. Maureen's journey of self-discovery continued to explore earlier themes, widening her awareness at her own pace and in her own time. Animals continued to figure strongly

(Maureen emphasised that she regarded the animals as friends). I felt that the importance Maureen attached to 'friendship' helped give her the strength to face a potentially difficult scene and issue. The animals, I think, offered her the support and comfort she needed, helping her develop a place of safety for Maureen — a place where she could explore death.

The fourth session

In the fourth and final session, I wanted to build on the safety already established so that Maureen could explore the rest of the story that still remained unexplored and hidden. I suggested to Maureen that she stage a scene in which she felt safe. She was a little dismayed that the image of the scene in her visualisation was exactly the same as in session three. I encouraged her to portray the scene using objects exactly as she had visualised them, as it seemed there might be some meaning in the duplicated scene. In a similar manner to the previous session, Maureen explored the objects and what they represented. I continued to encourage Maureen to repeat the process, even if she found the same meaning as the last time; Maureen felt she had discovered nothing about the scenario. I suggested that she might like to experiment with the scene and asked her to change the set as she wished, though I also assured her that she could return the set to its original form if she wished. Maureen removed one animal, then another. I checked how she felt, so as to keep working within the boundaries of her 'safety'. Maureen continued to remove over half the set, mostly the animals around the periphery of the scene. She felt happy with the new scene, and decided to make no further changes. She gave the scene the caption, 'The complete ending'.

Her caption suggested she had done what she needed to do, and had resolved some inner issue that had meaning for her. I felt the scene resembled a deathbed scene, the animals located around Jesus on the cross, Mary the mother of Christ, and the path (looking more like a coffin). The scene may have been a form of fiction, but it had the effect of producing a well-disguised masking of reality, perhaps the staging of Maureen's funeral.

Brook (1987) has explored the masks actors wear and how the masking of their faces consents to safety:

> [the mask] *gives you something to hide behind* [because it] *makes it unnecessary for you to hide. This is the fundamental paradox that exists in all acting: that because you are in safety, you can go into danger. It is very strange, but all theatre is based on that. Because there is a greater security, you can take greater risks; and because here it is not you, and therefore everything about you is hidden, you can let yourself appear.*

(Brook, 1987: 231)

Given that the animals were possibly symbols of friendship, removing them might have represented Maureen's readiness to leave the world of familiarity and loved ones and move towards her death (and therefore the unknown). She was able to face her own death indirectly from behind the mask of fiction.

Maureen may have expressed different meanings, both conscious and unconscious. I have tried to interpret some of these hidden meanings for the purpose of reflection. However, her own caption — 'The complete ending' — clearly stated she had completed a journey, and that she had found the necessary meaning to help her move forward. The scene possibly acted as a rehearsal, preparing Maureen for the day when she would have to say goodbye to her friends and pass away. The rehearsal, I believe, enabled her to process feelings under 'safe' conditions in which she was less likely to feel overwhelmed.

A separate space

I can only assume what Maureen's story might mean, based on my own observations and on the evidence that she had provided through her projections onto the objects, but she said herself that the work had given her the chance to explore issues she felt she needed to, without having to discuss them with friends and family. She felt she needed a 'separate space' where her loved ones were not 'polluted' by what she called a 'grim and depressing' subject.

Yalom (1985: 23) discusses the importance of exploring feelings about death so that life can be lived more fully: 'Dying often separates one from those to whom one is closest. One protects or cheers friends by an airy façade. Dying patients avoid morbid talk to such an extent that a wide gulf is created between them and the living'.

Through this therapeutic work, Maureen was able to give voice to her concerns, protecting her family and friends but addressing her needs to explore death, consequently bringing a new quality to her life. The space, the stage and the piece of paper enabled Maureen to explore issues in a safe way, whereby she could make connections through the objects and understand her circumstances in a way that made sense to her. Gersie (1996: 235) writes:

> *Symbolic expression, through painting, sound making, movement, drama or storytelling helps us to address our predicament in an indirect way, thereby gently easing our attempts to control the healing process.*

After the therapy, Maureen was a different patient to the patient I'd first met on the ward, laid in her bed feeling depressed. At the end of four sessions, she appeared bright, positive and full of hope. She was sat up on her bed fully clothed, and even her relatives had perceived a significant change in her outlook on life and on her circumstances.

Summary

A well-prepared ending enables us to face loss and feel present, rather then associating dying and death with separation and loneliness (Hinton, 1967: 27). A good ending helps contain our fears, offering safe engagement in a 'carefully designed process of closure'. A ritual ending acts as a framework to express feelings in a symbolic act that, according to Roose-Evans (1994: 5), can go 'deeper then words'. The ritual enabled Maureen, for example, to mark a significant transition in her life; it acted as a rite of passage, ending her journey and offering her 'permission to embark upon different journeys' (Gersie, 1991: 29). The scene offered her creative expression that generated a feeling of 'newness' and furthered her 'sense of mastery' (Gersie, 1991: 235) as she embarked on her journey towards the unknown.

However, ending is also a process of integrating reality by which, with appropriate support, people such as Maureen can process and reflect on their ending, and find new wisdom in dying.

A good ending prepares an individual for the impact of dying and death. It helps them create a process of closure by which they can safely integrate the reality and meaning of loss in their lives in order to move on. Maintaining honest and open communication of potentially powerful feelings in a safe and contained way helps facilitate, with respect, an individual's process of grief. A ritual that helps express and share what can be an inexpressible sense of loss 'sanctions' the separation that is required to embark on a new journey.

References

Brook P (1987) *The Shifting Point: 40 Years of Theatrical Exploration 1946–1987*. Methuen Drama, London

Clarkson P (1995) *The Therapeutic Relationship in Psychoanalysis, Counselling Psychology and Psychotherapy*. Whurr Publishers Ltd, London

Duggan M, Grainger R (1997) *Imagination, Identification and Catharsis in Theatre and Therapy*. Jessica Kingsley Publishers, London

Emunah R (1996) Five progressive phases in dramatherapy and their implications for brief dramatherapy. In: Gersie A (ed) *Dramatic Approaches to Brief Therapy*. Jessica Kingsley Publishers, London

Fransella, Dalton (2000) *Personal Construct Counselling in Action*. Sage, London

Gersie A (1991) *Storymaking in Bereavement: Dragons Flight in the Meadow*. Jessica Kingsley Publishers, London and Bristol, Pennsylvania

Gersie A (1996) Introduction. In: Gersie A (ed) *Dramatic Approaches to Brief Therapy*. Jessica Kingsley Publishers, London

Hinton J (1967) *Dying*. Penguin Books, England

Jennings S (ed) (1997) *Theory and Practice 3*. Routledge, London

Jewett C (1984) *Helping Children Cope with Separation and Loss*. Batsford, London

Kübler-Ross E (1970) *On Death and Dying*. Routledge, London

Mackay (1996) Brief dramatherapy and collective creation. In: Gersie A (ed)
    Dramatic Approaches to Brief Therapy. Jessica Kingsley Publishers, London

Parkes CM (1996) *Bereavement: Studies of Grief in Adult Life*. New edn. Penguin
    Books, London

Rinpoche S (1992) *The Tibetan Book of Living and Dying*. Rider Books, London

Roose-Evans (1994) *Passages of the Soul: Rediscovering the Importance of Rituals in
    Everyday Life*. Element, London

Wilson K, Kendrick P, Ryan U (1992) *Play Therapy: a Non-directive Approach for
    Children and Adolescents*. Balliere Tindall, London

Winnicot DW (1971) *Playing and Reality*. Penguin, Harmondsworth, Middlesex

Yalom ID (1980) *Existential Psychotherapy*. BasicBooks, USA

Yalom ID (1985) *The Theory and Practice of Group Psychotherapy*. 3rd edn.
    HarperCollins, USA

Chapter 8

Spirituality and social work in palliative care

Stephen R Everard

Introduction — what is spirituality?

Among authors and researchers, there seems to be no commonly agreed definition of the word 'spiritual'. Lloyd (1997), however, provides a useful starting point. In a study of people who were dying or bereaved, she defined spirituality as 'a dimension which brings together attitudes, beliefs, feelings and practices reaching beyond the wholly rational and material'.

A person's spirituality can include, or motivate a search for, that which is of 'ultimate' value as well as that which gives meaning or purpose to life. Many authors would include a reference to the 'transcendent', whether or not this is perceived in terms of a deity. Indeed, the 'spiritual' is often described as being expressed in terms of relationships — with God, with others, or with oneself. Dom (1999) talks of spirituality as being concerned with the 'transcendental, inspirational and existential way of living, as well as fundamentally and profoundly with the person as a human being, in relation to God and creation'.

At the same time, there is general agreement that a person's spirituality is different from, but may include or be related to, his or her religious belief. There also seems to be an overlap between spirituality and the psycho-emotional realm, although the two areas do not equate.

One question on which there is less agreement is whether the spiritual nature of a person is an aspect of the 'total' person, influencing and reacting to other aspects of that person (for example, the physical state or the sense of well-being) — or whether it is the integrating, synthesising component of the person, the 'animating... principal of the self' (Dickenson, 1975).

If pain is 'the result of conflict between a stimulus and the whole individual' (Leriche quoted by Saunders, 1988), spiritual pain can be similarly defined and manifested in, for example, a sense of separation from God or from others; a disruption in those relationships; a loss of meaning or purpose; and a searching for a resolution of these experiences — perhaps expressed in terms of anger, expressions of guilt, despair and withdrawal. Spiritual pain may be caused by an experience that completely shatters a person's view of life; which takes the meaning and focus out of their existence and leaves them desolate and helpless. O'Brien (1982; referenced in Dom, 1999) lists seven common human experiences under the general category of 'altered spiritual integrity': spiritual pain, alienation, anxiety, guilt, anger, loss and despair. Dom states that spiritual needs can broadly be categorised as: 'the need for love and harmonious relationships with humans, living entities and God; the need for forgiveness; the need for a source of hope and strength; the need for trust; the need for expression of personal beliefs and values; and the need for spiritual practice'.

Although not synonymous with spirituality, the part that institutional religion plays for some people should not be overlooked. Labun (1988) suggests that it 'codifies and provides pathways for the expression of belief and values held by the person. It provides meaning in the day to day choices of life and sustains the person through personal hardships such as illness, pain and personal disaster. It provides an avenue for celebrations when hardships are overcome'. The expression of spirituality is also shaped by the practices and beliefs of different cultures and by such a system as the family of upbringing.

For people who belong to a faith community, spirituality has a very specific set of defining principles that help people understand and make sense of their lives, including their most profound losses. 'If we are to accept that the spiritual aspect of a person is just as important as other aspects of our being, if not more so, we must pay attention to the beliefs, practices, rites and rituals that govern individuals' (Dom, 1999).

Spirituality in palliative care

The ego, a pauper in defence at the best of times, was quite baffled by the darkening spectre. Denial was the subterfuge of the meek and mild, hoping against hope, eking out their bleak anomic lives in whose penultimate phases they had already lost the little reason they had for living. Yet they could not look beyond their flickering spirits to stare at the shadows beyond. They spent their lives unthinking, as in most of their lives, and drifted into death with eyes averted, concerned with the immediate, and therefore bodily minutiae.

(Cappon, 1961)

Spiritual care has always been seen as an essential element of specialist palliative care, but its implementation and interpretation have changed over the years. Walter has identified three broad approaches to the theories and practice of spiritual care in palliative care through the years. As described by Cobb (2001), the first approach is that of the religious community, where faith is important and preparing for death is preparing for the life *beyond* death. The second is where there is no distinction between the spiritual and the religious, and the response to the presentation of spiritual issues is to refer patients to the chaplain. In the third approach, spiritual care is the responsibility of the multidisciplinary team 'because it concerns the human search for meaning which is applicable to everyone regardless of faith' (Cobb, 2001: 92).

With whatever approach, spiritual support is assumed to be a central part of the holistic care provided by specialist palliative care services. For example, the National Council for Hospice and Specialist Palliative Care Services, in its Occasional Paper 8, *Specialist Palliative Care: a Statement of Definitions*, states that one characteristic of a specialist palliative care service is that 'it provides physical, psychological, social and spiritual support, with a mix of skills, delivered through a multiprofessional, collaborative team approach'.

Suggesting that the spiritual care needs of patients and their families can be appropriately responded to by members of the multidisciplinary team raises questions of its own (see *Box 8.1*).

Box 8.1: Can the spiritual needs of patients and their families be met by the multidisciplinary team?

❖ To what extent are spiritual needs recognised and acknowledged within the institution?

❖ Are there identified members of the team to whom this care is entrusted, or is it assumed that such needs can be appropriately responded to by any member of the team?

❖ Are those, so entrusted, adequately trained, competent and confident tooffer such care?

❖ To whom are team members accountable for the care they give?

❖ Does the provision of spiritual care appear in job descriptions?

❖ Is there an agreed understanding within the institution of the meaning, focus and direction of spiritual care?

❖ Does the institution sufficiently nourish the reserves of compassion necessary to provide continual spiritual care?

❖ What, if any, expectations are generated of staff if spiritual care is advertised as being part of the multidisciplinary brief?

What do we mean by spiritual care? Price (2001) suggests that good spiritual care should be slow to intervene. She refers to Moore (1992), who says that to care for the soul, we need to undertake an 'observance' of it. Moore goes on, 'The "–serv" relates to in its linguistic origins to the shepherding of sheep' and suggests that to take care of the soul, we must 'watch where the soul grazes' and intervene only when there is danger.

There are a range of spiritual issues that might occur in a palliative care setting, including loss, suffering, a search for meaning, hope and religious belief. I will explore each in turn.

Loss

Loss is an integral aspect of dying: loss of function, loss of dignity, loss of independence and loss of identity. How a person sees himself or herself is a complex amalgam of factors. It includes a physical dimension (how we look, our ability to function, our sense of physical well-being); the roles we play in family life (husband, partner, parent, provider); and the roles we play in work and society (social worker, 'life and soul' of the party, golf-club captain, etc). Many or all of these dimensions are threatened and ultimately destroyed by a terminal illness. For some, it is the individual losses that are grieved for most: loss of hair, for example, or loss of libido. Some may be driven to ask deeper questions: who am I? And in relation to whom, or what? Having to face such questions, often brought on by a terminal illness, can trigger a crisis by which the individual's system of norms, values or beliefs is severely undermined. Moss (2002) suggests that it is the experience of loss, especially significant loss, that makes us question meanings we previously took for granted.

Suffering

Suffering is not synonymous with physical pain, though that is often an element within it. Even physical pain is experienced in different ways, according to how it is understood and the meaning invested in it. Pain can be part of a rewarding experience, such as the pain of an Olympic athlete striving for glory or a woman giving birth. It can also be a warning signal that stimulates action. Alternatively, it can be overwhelming and devastating, and have no perceived value at all.

Speck (1988) found that, in the early stages of their illness, people speak of 'pain', whereas later (with bone metastases, for example), they speak of 'suffering'. The word 'pain', he suggests, is used when it is easier to understand the message being given by the pain, and where there is hope of relief. The word 'suffering', on the other hand, is used to indicate decay and growing helplessness. Cassel (1982) describes suffering as occurring 'when an impending destruction of the person is perceived; it continues until the threat of disintegration has passed or until the integrity of the person can be restored in some other manner'. The context, as well as the intensity, of pain is relevant to the way it is experienced. This context contributes to the meaning of the pain for the individual, and therefore to the extent to which the pain is experienced as 'suffering'.

A person is made up of many 'parts', including their personality and character; their previous experiences and memories; their relationships; roles; and cultural background; as well as their activities, regular behaviours and perceived futures. The threat of 'impending destruction' can be made to any part of the person — for instance, to their normal activities (by deteriorating health); to their relationships (by no longer being able to function in that relationship as they did before); and to their perceived future (by a terminal illness).

Spiritual pain occurs when 'the meaning and focus of a person's existence is removed, leaving them desolate and helpless' (Dom, 1999). Saunders (1988) writes: 'The realisation that life is likely to end soon may well give rise to feelings of the unfairness of what is happening, and at much of what has gone before and, above all, a desolate feeling — of meaninglessness. Here lies, I believe, the essence of spiritual pain'.

Dom (1999), again, writes: 'It is important to recognise that there is a level of pain far deeper than the pain of a particular loss. The deeper pain is often associated with something totally destroyed at the centre of a person's being. This can be described as the person's view of life, their relationship with God, a map or picture of what life is about for them, or the values and principles they hold dear to their lives'.

Meaning

First, suffering is personal — that is, specific to the individuals concerned — and directly related to the meaning that person gives to the stimulus. Second, it is temporal, relating particularly to the person's perception of their future. Third, it is related to the degree of control a person feels able to exercise in response to the stimulus.

In our contemporary society, perhaps owing to increasing secularisation, the purpose of one's life has become associated with a search for self-identity, and there has been a growing identification of the self with the body. Some patients may deny that their condition is terminal and, in their eyes, meaning may be found in the fight for survival. Physical ill-health and the prospect of death, however, first threaten, then demolish this future-orientated, body-as-self construct. As Mellor and Shilling (1993) put it: '[when death occurs, the patients'] self-projects will be incomplete, their fragile attempt at personal meaning left shattered by the brute fact of death'. The threat that death brings to this understanding of self is meaninglessness: the shattering of an individual's sense of self and what is real. Thus, a key element of the experience of a terminal illness — for those with the capacity, consciously or unconsciously, to undertake it — is the search for meaning within it. Often, the search for meaning does not leave the physical level ('Why did he get cancer — he never smoked? If only the doctor had diagnosed it sooner...'). For many, the questions do not get asked at all, nor even thought, perhaps because the person is too busy feeling physically ill and is occupied with the task of coping with daily life. For some, the answers to these questions are sought at the moral level — 'Why me? I've lived a good life' — whereas, for others, the answer is sought in relation to a deity (the will of God, or the impact of a punishing God) or in the all-pervasive power of 'fate'.

Meaning is not just sought for the terminal condition, but for one's life as a whole — for 'what the last seventy years have added up to' (Lunn, 1993). Much of this search takes place in the past, reviewing one's life, looking at past relationships, accomplishments, and so on. But it may also be understood in terms of one's part in a greater 'scheme'.

Finding meaning does affect the experience of suffering. Cassell (1982) proposed that 'suffering is reduced when it can be located within a coherent set of meanings'. Kaczorowski (1989), from his study of spiritual well-being and anxiety in adults with cancer, concluded that 'meaning and purpose in life exceed a relationship with a higher being in relating to anxiety in some people'. Change in the experience of suffering is therefore possible. Saunders (1988) argued that an acceptance of mystery and of the inadequacy of human understanding leads patients to find unexpected resources and new self-awareness.

Through all of this, it is important to remember that palliative care includes not just the experience of the dying person, but also that of the family and carers, both before death and in bereavement. For them, physical suffering and loss will of course be smaller, but other suffering — the sense of loss, the search for meaning in the experience, and anxieties about the future — will be as great, if not greater. Their spiritual needs demand just as much attention.

Hope

Hope is a vital part of our personhood. In her study of people with a terminal illness, Herth (1990) found that hope was both dynamic and complex. Far from being tied to the aim of physical recovery, her study showed, hope is present at all stages of a terminal illness and even grows in the later stages of that illness. It is therefore a way of living with, even transcending, the dying process.

Herth defined hope as 'an inner power that facilitates the transcendence of the present situation and movement toward new awareness of enrichment of being'. She studied a sample group of terminally ill patients at different stages during what was understood to be their final six months of life. From the responses received from her sample, Herth proposed seven categories of hope-fostering strategies:

1. Interpersonal connectedness (being able to share in a meaningful relationship or 'being part of something').
2. Attainable aims (a purpose or sense of direction).

3. A 'spiritual base' (belief in God or a higher being; prayers; participation in religious activities; etc).
4. Personal attributes (determination, courage and serenity).
5. Lightheartedness.
6. Uplifting memories.
7. Affirmation of worth.

With respect to the attainable aims, it was noted that these were redefined and refocused as the patients deteriorated physically and their limitations became more evident. The experiences that were found to hinder hope fell into three categories: abandonment (by others) and isolation; uncontrollable pain; and devaluation of personhood.

The descriptions of hope given by the interviewees were stable across the three interview periods (when assessed at having a prognosis of six months or less; when severe impairment in their ability to complete activities of daily living were noted; and when their symptoms suggested that death would occur within two weeks). However, during the last two weeks, the only hope-fostering activities referred to fell within the categories of inter-personal connectedness, spiritual base and attainable aims. Yet the level of hope, as measured on an index formulated by Herth, actually increased during the final interview phase.

Age, sex, family income, education and fatigue levels did not appreciably affect the levels of hope. As for sources of hope, family, friends, healthcare professionals and God (or a higher being) were those most often identified.

Cousins (1979), quoted by Dom (1999), writes:

Death and dying are not the ultimate tragedy of life. The ultimate tragedy of life is depersonalisation: separation from spiritual nourishment that comes from being able to reach out to a loving hand, alienation from a desire to experience the things that make life worth living, separation from hope.

Religious belief

There is evidence that people with a religious faith that provides 'a meaning-endowing framework in terms of which all of life is understood' (Donahue, 1985), sometimes described as 'intrinsic faith', have less fear of death and more positive 'death attitudes' (Ellison, 1983; Kahow and Dunn, 1975). These people were more likely to have found their faith a help than those for whom their beliefs were more a matter of social convention. A belief in a positive life after death is also likely to be a help to people (Cartwright, 1991).

It is not, however, simply a question of whether people have a religious belief and how important that belief is to them. Smith *et al* (1983: 229) conclude that:

> *it is not the belief (in life after death) that is the most important determinant of death fear; it is rather the certainty with which that belief is held. Individuals who are close to death appear to derive comfort from a firm belief on one of two ends of a continuum. On the one end, there is a belief in a continued and rewarding existence after death. On the other, there is a belief in the finality of death. Those who are in the middle of this continuum, and who are most uncertain or ambivalent about what death brings, are also most fearful.*

Social work and spirituality

> *Holistic care involves an appreciation of the term 'spirituality' and the ability to respond effectively to the spiritual needs of the individual. Spiritual care aims to bring harmony and balance back into the life of the person suffering from a long-term illness.*

> (Dom, 1999)

The perception of the relation between the spiritual realm and social work has changed over the years. For many, entering the relatively new profession of social work had been a practical expression of deeply held beliefs. Yet, as social work sought to establish itself as a profession, it sought an academic foundation and a value base in which the spiritual, and certainly the language of religion, did not feature. One argument against the inclusion of a spiritual dimension in social work has been that it is esoteric and unobservable and should therefore play no part in a social science that seeks to be quantifiable and systematic. A second objection was the concern that the practitioner may impose his or her own spiritual or religious beliefs onto the client.

Recently, in the USA, however, there has been increasingly serious interest in the role of religion and spirituality in social work practice. Moss (2002) quotes a recent report from the Center For Policy On Aging in which Howse, the author of the report, 'points to a growing movement in the USA which recognises the health implications of spirituality and is trying to place responsibility for patients' religious care jointly between social care professionals and institutional religion... Some medical academics are even calling for spiritual needs assessments' (cited in *Community Care*, 4 November, 1999). There is, Moss says, little evidence at present of this interest being paralleled in social work training in the UK, although the CCETSW (Central Council for Education and Training in Social Work) made the following challenging statement:

> *Everyone is influenced by religion and religious practices whether*
> *they are believers, agnostics or atheists. Social service users are no*
> *exception. Yet religious and cultural practices, group and individual*
> *spirituality, religious divisions and religion as therapy, have had*
> *no place in social work education and practice... Ever the invisible*
> *presence in modern social work, its place should be recognised and*
> *taken account of in the work of the profession.*

(Patel et al in Moss, 2002).

Social work as practiced in palliative care is not a clearly defined phenomenon. The way the role is developed and the tasks expected of social workers differ from hospice to hospice for a variety of reasons, including how long the hospice has had social workers as members of their team; the source of funding of the social workers employed; and the qualifications, experience and skills of the post-holders (indeed, it is not unusual for social workers to be able to offer other qualified input to the multi-professional team, such as counselling and play therapy).

Social work in palliative care is also affected by the changes in delivery of health and social care — most notably, of late, those changes brought in following the National Health Service and Community Care Act (NHSCCA) (1990), with its 'mixed economy of welfare and the dominance of the language of consumerism' (Lloyd, 1990). Local authority social work, in particular, has become focused on regulation and the allocation of scarce resources in the assessment of risk and the completion of systematised and bureaucratic tasks.

Social workers in palliative care find themselves experiencing a fundamental clash of values as their rich, if short, heritage of client-focused work with patients and families meets the 'post-modern marketplace culture of health and welfare services' (Lloyd, 1990). Such a clash is felt, for example, when the work that social workers do with dying or bereaved people, which they adjudge to be of great importance, is given low priority or even squeezed out.

With respect to the relationship between social work and spirituality, social workers are increasingly working in situations of religious and cultural pluralism and must take into account the interplay of social, cultural, psychological and emotional factors for the individual. Yet Lloyd's research, referred to above, showed that a minimal number of social workers saw their role as including any spiritual care element, and only a few more identified helping clients with questions of meaning and peace, while a similarly small number identified themselves as having skills to explore the spiritual resources of the client.

However, about the distinguishing characteristics of work with people who are dying and bereaved (in the context of their work as a whole), the second most identified variable was existential issues (42%), and 12% identified 'spiritual or religious context'. Moreover, when focusing on the experiences of the dying or bereaved, 82% of the social workers asked thought that 'spiritual pain' was 'always', 'most times' or 'sometimes' present and 77% described the presence of 'philosophical questioning'.

In support of the need for spiritual issues to be given a central place in palliative care, it is significant that of the twenty-three dying or bereaved people interviewed, only one said he was without any form of belief system (and even he had found himself acknowledging a dimension that reached beyond the tangible and material). For the other twenty-two, religious and spiritual issues formed an integral part of their grief.

Assessment

A key part of any social work intervention is assessment. What kind of assessment is consistent with the provision of good spiritual care? If the 'spiritual' concerns the 'essence' of a person — that which makes them who they are — then the assessment process must be person-centred. In other words, it must be focused around the needs and wishes of the client. It must also allow the client the opportunity to dictate the agenda — to present to the assessor their own issues and concerns. It is unlikely (though by no means impossible) that this will happen in a single meeting, since the establishment of a trusting relationship rarely happens immediately and existential and spiritual issues related to death and dying seldom surface in time-limited dialogues.

To what extent is this kind of assessment possible in palliative care? It will depend largely on the nature of the referral to the social worker, but some aspects of the social work role will certainly make such an assessment difficult.

Care management

A referral to the social worker requesting the provision of a care package, to enable a patient to go home from hospital or hospice in-patient unit, often requires a rapid and task-focused assessment of need and resources. The agenda, although needs-related, is led by the social worker and shaped by the information needs of the organisation that will be providing the care. The social worker can handle the process compassionately, ensuring respect for the wishes of the patient and their carers; they can provide a voice for the client's wishes; they can involve the client as fully as they wish to be involved (eg. in discussions, in home assessment visits, in case conferences, etc) and ensure good communication with the client.

If the outcome meets the client's wishes (eg. the desire to spend last weeks at home, in familiar surroundings, accessible to family and friends), then the client's sense of well-being is likely to have been enhanced. Sadly, however, the motivation for the client to return home, or to move to a nursing home, does not always come from the client, but may be led by pressure from limited bed resources or from the patient being deemed not to require Specialist Palliative Care (because the needs of other patients are greater). A discharge process that does not emanate from, or accord with, the client's wishes is more likely to create spiritual difficulties than to be a medium for meeting spiritual needs.

Other practical work

Other practical social work in palliative care is more likely to be perceived by the patient and their family as being of benefit to them. Facilitating the receipt of appropriate State benefits or grants that will improve the patient's quality of life is likely to improve their sense of well-being, as will advocacy for improvements in housing or facilitating the making of a will. The recognition that the social worker has provided good practical care can also have a beneficial effect on the trust that the client then places in the worker, with the possibility that they may then confide issues that are more personally held.

Emotional work

Much of the work of palliative care social work lies within the realm of emotional support. Such work may be with the patient, or it may be with others affected by the illness — most often close family members or other carers. Referrals may be because of difficulties adjusting to the knowledge or impact of the illness; they may be for pre-bereavement support, as the family member anticipates the death and what life will be like without the patient; or they may relate to the impact of previous losses or life events on the ability to cope with the current life-threatening illness.

In this work, a trusting relationship needs to be established, with the social worker making himself or herself physically and emotionally 'present'. The social worker needs to be focused on the client, on their needs and wishes: 'It is the patient who is, or who should be, the centre. The question is his because it is his situation and he is the person who matters' (Saunders quoted in Pearson, 1969). We need to curb any inclination to decide what is best for the patient before fully understanding what the patient wants for himself or herself. We also need to avoid the desire to seek to refer on, too quickly, to an 'expert'. By so doing, an opportunity to provide spiritual support may be missed and may not come again. Being present when patients express their intimate thoughts and feelings provides the opportunity for affirmation and acceptance; challenges the isolation of suffering; and creates 'space' for meaning and growth.

Self-disclosure is important since there is evidence that carers' self-disclosure increases the likelihood of the clients doing the same (Dom, 1999). Social workers have to be prepared to lower their defensive barriers and open themselves up to their own vulnerability. By so doing, real contact can be made with clients. Sometimes, as de Hennezel (1998) says, 'showing someone we are helpless, deeply moved or vulnerable helps the patient to accept their human condition and the difficulty of their fate'.

Greater openness to such communication may feel uncomfortable for some social workers. Several of the social workers who responded to Lloyd's questionnaire commented that they would refer any questions or problems to do with faith to the appropriate religious minister or leader. On the face of it, this would seem a perfectly reasonable approach. However, for the person whose spiritual pain is experienced as an integral part of the complex mess of which they are trying to make some sense, such a response may not seem to meet their needs. Whilst the social worker would quite properly leave the control of physical pain to the doctor or nurse, he or she would continue to try to understand its impact and the significance of the physical aspects of the illness on the person's life as a whole. Similarly, appropriate referral to a religious leader should arise from sensitive exploration of the range of issues with which the dying or bereaved person is struggling, and should not preclude a continuing openness to such discussions.

Facilitating the expression of pain

As a relationship with a client develops, social workers may be in a position to facilitate the client's expression of pain, to help the client give voice to his or her feelings, be they feelings of anger, guilt, desperation, anxiety or sadness. The experience of loss can be palliated by reflective conversation. Articulating such thoughts and feelings can help patients through spiritual crises and contribute to some kind of resolution and acceptance. This may lead to an exploration of past memories and current fears, enabling both reflection and interpretation, which in turn can result in a greater sense of meaning and hope. What the social worker must avoid doing is referring the patient to 'someone who knows about these things' before the client has had a chance to express such thoughts and feelings. Their need is to express them now — and they have chosen you.

Who we are as carers becomes as important as what we know in determining the outcome of such meetings. The skill and humanity of the worker, no matter what professional role is being fulfilled, becomes just as important to the person in need as the practical out-workings of that professional expertise (Moss, 2002). There is a need for personal integrity, so that there is no discrepancy between our words and our 'being there'. We need to give consideration to our own needs and spirituality, and to be aware of our weak points and potential prejudices. We also need to look after ourselves — to cater for our own need for inner stability and calm.

Rituals

Rituals are present in all societies and allow people to deal with ambiguities of change and give them meaning.

(Cobb, 2001: 57)

Rituals enact meaning, express beliefs, evoke emotions, represent ideals; in other words, they make the invisible tangible through actions and words... [they] *express something of the significance of the relationships which have ended and also of the sense of loss... which exists because of the meaning we make of our own life and the lives of others.*

(Marris, 1986; quoted by Cobb, 2001)

Rituals in palliative care tend to be associated with the time after a death has occurred. However, in the sense that they can be distinguished from other, non-ritualised acts by, amongst other things, their 'gravity... context (the place and times they occur)... use of an established order... the means and content of their communication... and their efficacy' (Rappaport, 1999: 3), it could be argued that rituals permeate many areas of the palliative care process (eg. the initial assessment meeting, the admission process, etc).

For social workers, aspects of our work can be seen as rituals, in that their very processes and structures create order for the client. To agree with the client what you are going to do, to do it, and then to confirm what you have done, can make safe and relieve inherent anxiety.

In the more commonly understood meaning of the term 'ritual', social workers may have a role to play in events that serve some of the purposes described by Marris (see above). In my own hospice, times for remembrance and reflection, thanksgiving services, special events for Christmas, etc, all involve members of the social work department, sometimes in a position of leadership.

Conclusion

According to Liossi and Mystakidou (1997), patients who are likely to adapt to dying with the least distress include those who receive sensitive and caring social support; those who have found meaning in their lives and suffering; and those who are given the opportunity to exercise some control over their lives. Spiritual pain occurs when the meaning and focus of a person's life is lost, leaving the person desolate and helpless.

In focusing on the needs and wishes of their clients, in using their skills and experience to facilitate the expression of spiritual and emotional pain, and in being willing to enter at some level into the search for meaning in, and some resolution of, the suffering that patients and their families experience, social workers in palliative care settings make an important contribution to the meeting of the spiritual needs of their clients.

References

Cappon D (1961) The dying. *Psychiatr Q* **33**: 466–89

Cartwright A (1991) Is religion a help around the time of death? *Public Health* **105**: 79–87

Cassell EJ (1982) The nature of suffering and the goal of medicine. *N Engl J Med* **306**(11): 639–45

Cobb M (2001) *The Dying Soul: Spiritual Care at the End of Life.* Open University Press, Buckinghamshire

De Hennezel M (1998) Intimate distance. *Eur J Palliat Care* **5**(2): 56–9

Dickenson C (1975) The search for spiritual meaning. *Am J Nurs* **75**(10): 1789–94

Dom H (1999) Spiritual care, need and pain — recognition and response. *Eur J Palliat Care* **6**(3): 87–90

Donahue MJ (1985) Intrinsic and extrinsic religiousness: review and meta-analysis. *J Pers Soc Psychol* **48**: 400–19

Ellison CW (1983) Spiritual well-being: conceptualisation and measurement. *J Psychol Theol* **11**(4): 330–40

Herth K (1990) Fostering hope in terminally-ill people. *J Adv Nurs* **15**: 1250–9

Hinton J (1972) *Dying.* 2nd edition. Penguin, Harmondsworth

Kaczorowski JM (1989) Spiritual well-being and anxiety in adults diagnosed with cancer. *Hosp J* **5**(3): 105–16

Kahoe RD, Dunn RF (1975) The fear of death and religious attitudes and behaviour. *J Sci Stud Relig* **14**(4): 379–82

Labun E (1988) Spiritual care: an element in nursing care planning. *J Adv Nurs* **13**: 314–20

Liossi C, Mystakidou K (1997) Heron's theory of human needs in palliative care. *Eur J Palliat Care* **4**(1): 32–5

Lunn L (1993) Spiritual concerns in palliation. In: Saunders C, Sykes N (eds) *The Management of Terminal Malignant Disease*. 3rd edn. Edward Arnold, London

Lloyd M (1997) Dying and bereavement, spirituality and social work in a market economy of welfare. *Br J Soc Work* **27**: 175–90

Mellor PA, Schilling C (1993) Modernity, self-identity and the sequestration of death *Sociology* **27**(3) 411–31

Moore T (1992) *Care of the Soul*. HarperCollins, New York

Moss B (2002) Spirituality: a personal perspective. In: Thompson N (ed) *Loss and Grief: a Guide for Human Service Practitioners*. Palgrave, London

National Council for Hospice and Specialist Palliative Care Services (1995) *Occasional Paper 8: 'Specialist Palliative Care: a Statement of Definitions'*

Pearson L (ed) (1969) *Death and Dying: Current Issues in Treatment of the Dying Person*. Case Western Reserve UP, Cleveland

Price S (2001) Has something changed? Social work, pastoral care, spiritual counselling and palliative care. *Prog Palliat Care* **9**(6): 244–6

Saunders C (1988) *Spiritual Pain*. AG Bishop & Sons Ltd (originally published in *Hospital Chaplain* **102**: 30)

Smith DK, Nehemkis AM, Charter RA (1983) Fear of death, death attitudes and religious conviction in the terminally ill. *Int J Psychiatry Med* **13**(3): 221–32

Speck P (1988) *Being There: Pastoral Care in Terminal Illness*. SPCK, London

Chapter 9

Social work and palliative care for people with dementia

Jonathan Parker

Introduction

> Lavinia Dawson had been diagnosed with Alzheimer's disease seven years before being admitted to a nursing home. Her husband, Frank, said regretfully that he could no longer cope with the physical strain of attending to her personal needs. He was emotionally drained, but did not say so. Their daughter, Jane, was relieved that her mother was now 'being looked after' and suggested to Frank that he could now have a 'well-earned rest' and that she would not know if he had visited or not, so he should leave it to the professionals. Frank was relieved but felt guilty because he could no longer look after Lavinia. The nursing attended to her physical needs, ensured that Frank did not know how disorientated and confused Lavinia had become, hoping not to upset him. When Lavinia contracted bronchopneumonia and it was clear she was unlikely to survive, they assured him it was a 'blessed relief'. People were sympathetic, but did not really understand why Frank was so distraught when Lavinia died.

Unfortunately, cases such as that of Lavinia are far from uncommon. Everyone involved was undoubtedly acting to protect Frank from pain and distress, but did so in a way that unwittingly deprived him of control, and devalued both Lavinia's remaining life and the life that she and Frank shared together.

In this chapter, we will examine the importance of palliative care social work practice for people who have dementia, and for their carers. Case-study material will provide an insight into the complex, demanding and central role that social workers can have in working in palliative care settings with people with dementia.

It is important to understand what we mean by the term 'dementia'; the various types of dementia; whom it affects; and how common it is. After examining definitions and meanings, this chapter will consider why social workers are involved in palliative care social work with people with dementia, and examine some of the literature concerning palliative care and dementia, which tends to exclude social work. The chapter will explore the importance of person-centred approaches to dementia care, and the emphasis on person-centred care in the National Service Framework for Older People (Department of Health [DoH], 2000). How this can influence and direct social work practice in the care-management of people with dementia at the end of life will also be considered. The chapter will go on to cover specific aspects of specialist social work with people with dementia and their carers, including bereavement issues and moves towards interdisciplinary and interprofessional working.

What is dementia?

It is commonly thought that dementia affects only the old. As a result, social work with people with dementia has been as marginalised in society as older people themselves (Martin and Bartlett, 2003; Parker and Penhale, 1998). However, we know that dementia affects people of all ages (Parsons, 2003), although it is more common in older people than in younger people (*Table 9.1*). If we are to understand palliative care and loss-focused social work with people with dementia, we need to consider what is meant by the term 'dementia'; how common it is; and whom it affects.

Table 9.1: Prevalence of dementia by age	
Age in years	**Prevalence**
40–65	1 in 1000
65+	1 in 50
70+	1 in 20
80+	1 in 5
90+	1 in 2

Source: Alzheimer's Society (2004).

Traditionally, dementia has been associated with biomedical neuropathological conditions resulting in a progressive decline in the global functioning of the indi vidual. Deterioration is physical, cognitive and social, a concept that underpins biomedical thought and practice (Royal College of Physicians, 1981). To understand dementia in this way represents a failure of medical practice founded on a curative approach (Parker, 2001), but it is perhaps indicative of moves towards including dementia care within palliative care and palliative medicine. However, dementia can also be understood as a subjectively experienced process in which the individuals gradually lose their 'moorings' to the familiar (Sabat and Harré, 1992; Cheston and Bender, 1999; Adams and Barlett, 2003). It is in this sense that Kitwood (1997) and Kitwood and Bredin (1992) articulated a socially constructed understanding of dementia as a process by which impairment and decline result from the interaction between the individuals, their neuropathology and the resulting treatment by others who interpret 'dementia' and associate it with particularly negative situations.

The interactive understanding of dementia is similar to the social model of disability (Oliver, 1990), in which it is not the impairment itself that disables but the way society operates in relation to that impairment. For social workers, understanding dementia as wider than the disease is central to working with the individual as a person, with the attendant psychological, social, physical and spiritual needs of each individual. It does not negate biomedical approaches and the search for treatments, but sees each experience of dementia as unique to the individual with dementia and his or her family, friends and social networks. It also understands that the care practices in which we engage contribute to the advancement of the dementia and its negative effects or the well-being of the person with dementia and those around them (Parker, 2003).

There are many different types of disease leading to dementia, the most common being dementias of the Alzheimer's type, vascular dementias and Lewy-body dementias. Whilst each type has a specific neuropathology and course, there are some differences in the impact on a person's personality, behavioural, cognition, emotion and physical health. Individual factors also influence the way a dementia is experienced. Social workers need a basic understanding of the types of dementia and the particular features associated with each one. Such understanding would help them deal with other professionals and with carers who are often immersed in biomedical understandings of dementia. Even more than this, however, they need to see the uniqueness of the individual and to consider the life, experiences and personality of the person and the influence of family, friends and other significant networks, ensuring that the person is not lost within the assumptions of decline, deterioration and death.

Although not a 'disease of old age', the likelihood of dementia rises with increasing age, with one in five people over eighty years having some degree of dementia (*Table 9.1*). Although this statistic may indicate a great concern for developing appropriate care and treatments, and economic considerations given the changing demography of the UK (*Table 9.2, Table 9.3*), it is heartening if interpreted in another way: about four in five people do *not* develop dementia, even at eighty years and above. It is important that social workers are aware of such statistics, which can help them in their work.

Of course, family caregivers may express questions of 'contractibility' and 'inheritance'. Social workers are not medically trained and not in a position to offer advice of a medical nature. However, it is important that they have some awareness of possible causation in order to present an informed perspective and to facilitate decision-making and choices amongst carers (Marriott, 2003).

Like all human beings, people with dementia eventually die. There are some who die as a result of some other condition; some who die of a complex mix of mental and physical problems, but for whom the dementia is not as advanced; and some who die as a result of complications of the dementia itself (Cox and Cook, 2003). In light of this, it is important to consider palliative care for people with dementia.

Table 9.2: Numbers of people with dementia in UK countries	
UK country	**Number of people with dementia**
England	634,000
Scotland	60,600
Northern Ireland	14,900
Wales	40,600
Total	**750,100**

Source: Alzheimer's Society (2004).

Table 9.3: Numbers of people of State-pensionable age in the UK	
Year	**Number in millions (actual/projected)**
2002	10.9
2011	12.2
2021	12.7
2031	15
2061	17

Source: UK Populations Projections (2003).

Palliative care and dementia

Demographic changes in the UK indicate that the numbers of older people with dementia will increase over the coming decades (*Table 9.2, Table 9.3*). There is a need for care services to be developed to support people with dementia and their family carers. However, at the present time, whilst the need to encompass a wider range of terminal illnesses is recognised, palliative care services often remain cancer-focused (Addington-Hall, 1998, 2000; Seymour and Hanson, 2001). This concentration on 'a select few' has led to other services being cut and provision for people dying in non-specialist resources, or not receiving palliative care services, being diminished (Seymour and Hanson, 2001). Studies of care delivery for people caring for older people in the last year of life show poor service coordination, communication problems between service providers and service users, and a lack of practical, emotional and social support for family carers.

These difficulties were reflected in Seymour and Hanson's (2001) study of nine chronically ill older people and nine family carers. Participants in the study indicated that they were not contacted by services unless carers sought them out; that planning and evaluation of care were lacking; and that there was an impression given that 'nothing more could be done'. Few specialist palliative care services include people with end-stage dementia (de Vries, 2003), although the focus on cancer is being challenged (ten Have and Clark, 2002).

Older people are generally less well-served in social care than younger people. This has been fuelled by the health and social care debate. The Royal Commission on Long Term Care (Sutherland, 1999) reports these tensions clearly, pointing out that health care is free at the point of need, whilst social care is means-tested. This could have particular implications for people with dementia who may receive social services care and be charged for it, as opposed to people with cancer or heart disease whose healthcare needs will be met at no cost to the recipient. This situation is increasingly recognised. One of the projects being carried out under the DoH's Older People and their Use of Services programme (OPUS) concerns the ways in which nursing professionals assist in the decision-making process about transition from curative to palliative care in non-cancer patients. In respect of dementia and palliative care, however, there are few studies published. McCarthy *et al* (1997) found that physical symptoms, pain management and types of services available differed for people with dementia compared with those dying of heart disease and cancers.

Palliative care itself considers the 'total care' of the person (Clark and Seymour, 1999), concerning the range of people's needs and meeting these in a multidisciplinary way. Indeed, the World Health Organisation (WHO) (1990) definition is important when expanding the concept to dementia care. The definition accepts death as a natural process whilst affirming life. It states that palliative care should:

- neither postpone nor hasten death
- provide relief from pain and distressing symptoms
- include spiritual and psychological care as well as physical care
- offer support during the patient's illness and post-bereavement.

The educational needs of staff are highlighted here and an understanding of palliative care issues and philosophies is important. Palliative care and hospice care can be understood as forming a philosophy of holistic care. It has only recently been recognised in the UK that the diseases causing dementia are terminal illnesses (de Vries, 2003). Whilst hospice or palliative care emphasises quality of life issues rather than the curative approach to medicine, the experience of the dying person with dementia has been largely ignored (Casarett and Karlawish, 1999; Cox and Cook, 2002).

The literature that exists in respect to dementia and palliative care tends to focus on nursing and medical needs such as mobility, problems with activities of daily living (ADLs), developing treatment guidelines (Lloyd-Williams and

Payne, 2002) and behavioural issues (Cox and Cook, 2002). The importance of this focus cannot be denied, especially since death often results from a secondary illness such as respiratory infection or another superimposed terminal illness such as cancer. However, as de Vries (2003) points out, there are increased ethical issues surrounding (re-)hydration or percutaneous endoscopic gastronomy feeding in people who find it difficult to communicate or make decisions (see also: Finucane *et al*, 1999; Billings, 2000; ten Have and Janssens, 2002). The argument for the palliative care approach to be widened is strengthened given that the need for familiarity, prevention of confusion and pain control are often indicated in people with dementia. The importance of pain-management and introducing the concepts of hospice for people with dementia is acknowledged as part of the range of their health and social work needs (Cox, 1996; Marshall, 2001; Evans, 2002).

The social, emotional, spiritual and psychological needs of the person translate into social work practice, as well as informing good nursing and medical practice in palliative care. For instance, recognising that people with dementia and their families may need assistance in staying together and in preserving routine if the patient is hospitalised, is important.

Why are social workers' involved with people with dementia?

Ever since the development of a care-management approach in the early 1990s, social workers have been involved with people with dementia and their families in an assessment capacity, looking at needs defined by a consumerist and bureaucratic model, as opposed to a holistic-care model. The over-rigid application of this approach has been criticised by Tibbs (2001).

Social workers are skilled in assessing need, act as managers and coordinators of care, and take a social and family perspective; they therefore work with people and their experiences of loss. As the Single Assessment Process is developed across health and social care, social workers can use their knowledge and skills to facilitate the sharing of best practice in coordinating services. The development of a more standardised set of eligibility criteria will assist in determining social work involvement in coordinating care where there is an inability to carry out vital tasks or these are substantially impaired (DoH, 2002) However, social workers must be wary of assuming a monopoly of skill in assessment and remember that effective palliative care for people with dementia relies on a multidisciplinary and multiprofessional approach, especially with respect to care planning. As de Vries (2003: 118) states from a nursing perspective:

When making decisions regarding medical or nursing interventions, individuals' own views and their wishes prior to dementia should, if known, be considered and the wishes of the family and recommendations of the multidisciplinary team should be taken into account.

Not all social workers work in statutory care management settings: social workers work in specialist teams, carrying out wider functions than the assessment of needs; they work in specific agencies dealing with dementia, in voluntary and independent settings, as well as statutory ones.

One specific locus for social work is within a hospice setting. Although few people with dementia also receive hospice care, this does happen.

Gertrude James was admitted to her local hospice for respite care. She had metastases from breast cancer, and had been diagnosed with dementia three years before developing cancer. Staff on the respite unit called the social worker because of her dementia, to discuss how, as a team, her care should be managed given her 'confusion and inability to communicate'. Whilst the situation was little different to many others experienced, the diagnosis of dementia raised anxieties. The social worker was, because of her role, able to spend time sitting with Gertrude and her relatives when they visited, getting to know her as she is now, her past life, interests and preferences. Although Gertrude was severely cognitively impaired, the social worker was able to pass on vital information from the family and from her observations of Gertrude, to assist nursing staff in their approach and delivery of appropriate care and to lessen anxieties resulting from the diagnosis of dementia.

There is an increasing emphasis on interdisciplinary and interprofessional approaches to health and social care. Interdisciplinary approaches may concern working between those who assess, those who coordinate, and those who deliver the care or support. Interprofessional approaches concern the ways in which social workers practise alongside nurses, therapeutic staff, GPs and medical practitioners (see *Chapter 4*).

Communication skills are a central part of the health and social work agenda for education (see *Chapter 6*). Social workers are able to use their understanding of communication issues with people with dementia, seeking creative and alternative ways of helping people communicate (Parker, 2003). This may take the form of observing preferences, gaining information about pasts likes and dislikes, and about preferred ways of doing things from family members and friends (Allan, 2001). In communicating directly with the person with dementia, the social worker needs to deploy listening skills that are sensitive to the whole person and the way they convey information, attending not only to the spoken words or sounds but also to emotions and body language. Often, when conversation is difficult or not possible, people with dementia can communicate using pictures, photographs and images. Being creative and genuinely committed to communication is central.

It is not always possible to determine when a person is in pain, but developing communication skills in health and social care can help. Information-sharing between professionals is crucial in ensuring that a person's needs are met and their preferences and wishes taken into account. Communication is vital to the success of the Single Assessment Process and ways to meet the needs of service users and carers must not be knocked off centre by an over-rigid use of data-protection legislation. Questions of confidentiality have taxed healthcare practitioners and social workers for many years. Studies have indicated that service coordination has often been lacking in providing care to older people with palliative care needs. The modernising agenda, in which health and social care agencies are able to pool budgets more easily and the Single Assessment Process is championed by the National Service Framework for Older People (DoH, 2002), help to ensure that information that needs to be known can be transferred to those who need to know it.

Social workers bring a particular and crucial perspective to health and social care delivery. They take an ecological and social approach, seeing the person in context. This means that, in making an assessment, the social worker considers the impact of the situation and the strengths and needs of others involved. For social workers practising in non-care-management settings, work with the wider family and friendship networks is central in developing ways for needs to be met.

Development of the person-centred approach to care and care-management social work

There has been a negative view of dementia, for instance, as a 'living death' (Woods, 1989; Parsons, 2001), that may have contributed to the devaluation of people with dementia and the patchy development of services. The development and gradual acceptance of social-disability models — which see the person in context affected by social and physical barriers erected against them and a personhood approach that emphasises dignity and respect, equal worth as human beings, and valuable biographies and preferences — bring a potential change to the construction and delivery of care services (Cox and Cook, 2002). These accord well with social work values and ethics.

Since the late 1980s onwards, a shift has taken place in the culture of care for people with dementia. Stemming from the commitment of the late Tom Kitwood — the psychologist and academic who championed person-centred and relational care for people with dementia — an approach developed that recognised that the process of dementia resulted not only from the neurological impairment of the individual, but also from the ways in which they were treated as individuals. This perspective could be extended to the effects of broader societal attitudes to ageing, ill-health and disability. In contemporary UK society, the end of life is a taboo subject.

Person-centred care is based on a process of respect for the person as an individual who is valued for themselves, their experiences in the past and the present, and their capacity for a future. Cox and Cook (2002: 99) see the merger of person-centred care and hospice or palliative care as fundamental in developing good end-of-life care for people with dementia:

> *In extending the person-centred approach of dementia care to those who are dying, care staff are more likely to understand and respond to pain, discomfort and difficult behaviour by trying to understand the person's behaviour as a means of communication. By drawing on expertise developed in specialist palliative care, staff can develop skills and knowledge of caring that are appropriate and so augment the knowledge already gained in looking after people with dementia.*

Parsons (2001: 131) recognises the importance of social workers assisting carers at the end-stage of life when people may have become more frail and dependent and need significantly increased care. Often, she points out, relatives may have already experienced a range of losses and social workers can assist in focusing on the person's pre-morbid wishes and values in planning and delivering care:

> *Identifying when a person has entered the final stage of dying with dementia is difficult for formal and informal carers who may for some time have regarded their relative as 'already dead' or 'as good as dead'. Hence such 'social death' preceded clinical or biological death... working alongside informal carers to enable them to continue caring for as long as they want to demands skill, creativity and cultural awareness. Community professionals and care staff need to ensure that a person's values are integrated into the process of dying.*

In considering the wishes and preferences of the person with dementia and the increasing interest in advanced directives and discussions of voluntary euthanasia, social workers have a moral responsibility to become directly involved in these debates. The Assisted Dying for the Terminally Ill bill, even if it were to become law, would preclude people with impaired decision-making capacity, such as people with dementia, from assisted suicide.

However, the Mental Incapacity Bill (2003, ss 23–25) would allow people to formulate advanced directives on the refusal of treatment at some point in the future. Social workers practise with a perspective that is wider than the individual and must grapple with the interpersonal and social implications of euthanasia and assisted suicide. Leichentritt's (2002) phenomenological study of the experiences, attitudes and meanings of sixteen Israeli social workers to various forms of euthanasia found a distinction between 'passive euthanasia' (the withholding or withdrawing of treatments that might sustain life) and 'active euthanasia' and assisted suicide (such as the administration of a death-hastening drug). A need for education programmes dealing with these issues was indicated. Social workers in palliative care settings have a clear role in facilitating discussion of these issues between professionals and listening to the perspectives of service users where possible and care-givers where appropriate.

Bereavement issues and dementia care

Bereavement in dementia has attracted some comment. There is, as we have seen, a sense of anticipated, then realised, loss. Indeed, in the USA, the term 'living bereavement' has been used to describe caregivers' experiences of looking after someone with dementia. The loss relates to the loss of personality, time together, functioning and a 'known other' in the life of the carer. These losses are experienced while the physical presence of the person remains.

There are many criticisms of this understanding of dementia, but the experiences of family carers may reflect a need for supportive social work and bereavement-type work as the following case shows:

> Peter Mason was wracked with guilt about his feelings concerning his wife, Lily. Lily Mason had had dementia since a stroke seven years before. Physically, she had been weakened, but her comprehension, ability to speak and recognition of familiar settings and people were also severely diminished. When it became clear that she was suffering from heart failure from which she would not survive, Peter said he felt very little — not even relief. He could not explain this reaction, other than to say that he had lost Lily many years ago, and that his care for her was out of respect to her memory. The social worker listened to Peter, allowed him to tell his story and affirm his past care without judging him.

At the end-stage of life, social workers can play an important part in contributing to the management of bereavement, in working with the bereaved family, and in normalising some of the ambivalence that might be felt. For social workers in care-management positions, it is likely that involvement will cease after bereavement (Tibbs, 2001), but social workers have an information-giving and advisory role that demands a knowledge of services and support available in the local area (Payne, 1995; MacDonald, 1999).

The needs of families and other carers do not just evaporate, and social workers and bereavement services in hospice settings are ideally placed to offer support. Often, people caring for someone with dementia will have done so for some time. It may be that some 'anticipatory' work has taken place. 'Anticipatory grief', a contested concept, is rather a reaction to losses brought about as a result of the illness, as opposed to an anticipation and working through of the prospective death of the individual (Currer, 2001). Dementia, especially Alzheimer's disease, has been linked to 'social death' or 'living bereavement', but grieving before the physical death of the individual may be more of a response to loss of status, social and emotional life, ambitions and economic security resulting from the dementia, than anticipatory grief.

Walker and Pomeroy (1996) regard this grieving for losses that have already taken place as being intimately linked with the depressive symptoms often experienced by carers. If so, it suggests that community services can be targeted to meet these needs, to work with grief and facilitate its expression rather than focus on the bereavement to come.

Payne, Horn and Relf (1999) point out, importantly, that not all post-bereavement changes are negative for carers and some people can draw on personal 'hardiness' or resilience. There may also be a degree of ambiguity relating to the experience: 'if they have been engaged in the long-term care of the deceased, such as in Alzheimer's disease, they no longer have those physical and emotional demands' (Payne *et al*, 1999: 33).

Depuis (2002) studied ambiguous loss and dementia care in adult children caring for people with dementia in long-term care. Her work suggests that the loss process moves through phases of anticipation, progressive realisation and acknowledgement, and that the degree of ambiguity shifts with time. The end result of dementia is death, and issues for the carers while the person with dementia is still alive may concern anticipation and even wishing to hasten the death of the person. These are significant aspects to be dealt with. After the death, there may be a need for social work involvement and bereavement support. Some of the issues are brought out in respect of Marilyn's family:

After Marilyn's death, at forty-eight years old, from a transmissible form of dementia, the hospice social worker who also coordinated the bereavement services was asked to support her two sons, Martin aged twelve and John aged nine. In the final few months of Marilyn's life, the boys had withdrawn from discussing the situation and, following her death, Martin said he felt no emotion at all, whilst John became very angry and volatile. James, the boys' father, expressed concern that they were not dealing with their mother's death, but stated quickly that he was fine.

The social worker was able to offer time to Martin and John, to find ways in which they could express themselves, in drawing, story-telling and making models, and to assure them that their feelings — ambiguous, hidden or expressed — were okay. At the same time, contact with the children allowed James to be more confident in stating his needs and upset at the bereavement.

It is also important for social workers to recognise bereavement and loss issues in the person with dementia and to develop communication skills that facilitate the exploration of these issues when a person may be severely cognitively impaired and unable to express or comprehend as before (Allan, 2001; Parker, 2003). Social workers, however, are instrumental in the move into residential care and need to understand, listen and assist with some of the loss and confusion that can arise from such a transition.

The skills involved in working with loss will translate from setting to setting and person to person. However, understanding the need to work with loss before death, after death and with the experiences of the person with dementia, demands particular knowledge and skills that call for education of social workers in palliative care and long-term dementia care settings.

Summary

Palliative care for people with dementia is generally lacking in the UK, but individual and family concerns indicate a considerable need, and certainly a wish, to integrate the principles of hospice when working with people with dementia in the later stages of life. The wider ecological and contextual perspectives taken by social workers provide a valuable focus for palliative care services for people with dementia. As the population of the UK ages, and more people are diagnosed with and live with dementia, the need for hospice and palliative care services will increase. Social work must play a central part in these services if appropriate person-centred and person-in-context approaches to care are to be developed.

References

Adams T, Bartlett R (2003) Constructing dementia. In: Adams T, Manthorpe J (eds) *Dementia Care*. Arnold, London

Addington-Hall J (1998) *Reaching Out: Specialist Palliative Care for Adults with Non-Malignant Diseases*. Occasional Paper 14. National Council for Hospice and Specialist Palliative Care and Scottish Partnership Agency for Palliative Cancer Care, London

Addington-Hall J (2000) *Positive Partnerships: Palliative Care for Adults with Severe Mental Health Problems*. Occasional Paper 17. National Council for Hospice and Specialist Palliative Care and Scottish Partnership Agency for Palliative Cancer Care, London

Allan K (2001) *Communication and Consultation: Exploring Ways for Staff to Involve People with Dementia in Developing Services.* Policy Press/Joseph Rowntree Foundation, Bristol

Alzheimer's Society (2004) Facts about Dementia. http://www.alzheimers.org. uk/Facts_about_dementia/Statistics/index.htm

Billings A (2000) Recent advances: palliative care. *BMJ* **321**: 555–8

Casarett D, Karlawish J (1999) *Working in the Dark: the State of Palliative Care for Patients with Severe Dementia.* Generations, Spring

Cheston R, Bender M (1999) *Understanding Dementia: the Man with the Worried Eyes.* Jessica Kingsley Publishers, London

Clark D, Seymour J (1999) *Reflections on Palliative Care.* Open University Press, Buckingham

Cox S (1996) Quality care for the dying person with dementia. *J Dementia Care* **July/ Aug**: 19–21

Cox S, Cook A (2002) Caring for people with dementia at the end of life. In: Hockley J, Clark D (eds) *Palliative Care for Older People in Care Homes.* Open University Press, Buckingham

Currer C (2001) *Responding to Grief: Dying, Bereavement and Social Care.* Palgrave, Basingstoke

DoH (2000) *National Service Framework for Older People.* DoH, London

DoH (2002) The Single Assessment Process: Guidance for Local Implementation. http://www.doh.gov.uk/scg/sap/locimp.htm

de Vries K (2003) Palliative care for people with dementia. In: Adams T, Manthorpe J (eds) *Dementia Care.* Arnold, London

Depuis S (2002) Understanding ambiguous loss in the context of dementia care: adult children's perspectives. *J Gerontol Soc Work* **37**(2): 93–115

Evans B (2002) Improving palliative care in the nursing home: from a dementia perspective. *J Hospice Palliat Care* **4**(2): 91–9

Finucane T, Christmas C, Travis K (1999) Tube feeding in patients with advanced dementia: a review of the evidence. *JAMA* **282**(14): 1365–70

Kitwood T, Bredin K (1992) Toward a theory of dementia care: personhood and well-being. *Ageing Soc* **12**: 269–87

Kitwood T (1997) *Dementia Reconsidered: the Person Comes First.* Open University Press, Buckingham

Leichtentritt R (2002) Euthanasia: Israeli social workers' experiences, attitudes and meanings. *Br J Soc Work* **32**(4): 397–413

Lloyd-Williams M, Payne S (2002) Can multidisciplinary guidelines improve the palliation of symptoms in the terminal phase of dementia? *Int J Palliat Nurs* **8**(8): 370–5

MacDonald A (1999) *Understanding Community Care.* Palgrave, Basingstoke

Marriott A (2003) Helping families cope with dementia. In: Adams T, Manthorpe J (eds) *Dementia Care.* Arnold, London

Marshall M (2001) Care settings and the care environment. In: Cantley C (ed) *A Handbook of Dementia Care.* Open University Press, Buckingham

Martin W, Bartlett H (2003) Valuing people with dementia. In: Adams T, Manthorpe J (eds) *Dementia Care*. Arnold, London

McCarthy M, Addington-Hall J, Altman D (1997) The experience of dying with dementia: a retrospective study. *Int J Geriat Psychiat* **12**: 404–9

Oliver M (1990) *The Politics of Disablement*. Macmillan, Basingstoke

Parker J (2001) Interrogating person-centred dementia care in social work and social care. *J Soc Work* **1**: 329–45

Parker J (2003) Positive communication with people who have dementia. In: Adams T, Manthorpe J (eds) *Dementia Care*. Arnold, London

Parker J, Penhale B (1998) *Forgotten People: Positive Approaches to Dementia Care*. Ashgate, Aldershot

Parsons M (2001) Living at home. In: Cantley C (ed) *A Handbook of Dementia Care*. Open University Press, Buckingham

Parsons M (2003) Living at home. In: Cantley C (ed) *A Handbook of Dementia Care*. 2nd edition. Open University Press, Buckingham

Payne M (1995) *Social Work and Community Care*. Macmillan, Buckingham

Payne S, Horn S, Relf M (1999) *Loss and Bereavement*. Open University Press, Buckingham

Royal College of Physicians (1981) Organic memory impairment in the elderly: implications for research, education and the provision of services. *J R Coll Physicians* **15**: 11–67

Sabat SR, Harre R (1992) The construction and deconstruction of self in Alzheimer's disease. *Ageing Soc* **12:** 443–61

Seymour J, Hanson E (2001) Palliative care and older people. In: Nolan M, Davies S, Grant G (eds) *Working with Older People and their Families: Key Issues in Policy and Practice*. Open University Press, Buckingham

Sutherland S (1999) *With Respect to Old Age: Long Term Care, Rights and Responsibilities: a Report by the Royal Commission on Long Term Care*. Cmnd 4192. HMSO, London

ten Have H, Clark D (eds) (2002) *The Ethics of Palliative Care*. Open University Press, Buckingham

ten Have, Janssens J (2002) Futility, limits and palliative care. In: ten Have H, Clark D (eds) (2002) *The Ethics of Palliative Care*. Open University Press, Buckingham

Tibbs M (2001) *Social Work and Dementia: Good Practice and Care Management*. Jessica Kingsley Publisher, London

UK Population Projections (2003) http://wwww.statitics.gov.uk/pdfdir/pop1203.pdf

Walker R, Pomeroy E (1996) Depression or grief: the experiences of caregiving of people with dementia. *Health Soc Work* **21**(4): 247–54

Woods R (1989) *Alzheimer's Disease: Coping with a Living Death*. Souvenir Press, London

WHO (1990) *Cancer Pain Relief and Palliative Care*. Technical Report Series No. 804. WHO, Geneva

Chapter 10

Specialist palliative care social work with people who have learning disabilities

Linda McEnhill

Introduction

This chapter will outline some key areas in the development of practice with a client group that has previously been greatly neglected in palliative care research and literature. By drawing on the shared practice of colleagues and the lived experience of clients, I hope to stimulate debate and creative thinking in this crucial area of care.

Case study: David's story

David was a middle-aged, moderately learning-disabled man living in a residential service when he was diagnosed with the recurrence of a brain tumour. When the tumour was first diagnosed, it was thought to be secondary to another malignancy in his body which was not found. David underwent surgery and although not all of the tumour could be removed, no follow-up (oncology) treatment was offered on the basis of his 'pre-morbid condition' — ie. his learning disability and mental health problems. Consequently, the diagnosis of recurrence was experienced by David, and those that cared for him, as a death sentence.

Definitions of 'learning disability'

Learning disability is a condition that exists from childhood and includes the presence of significant intellectual impairment and deficits in social functioning or adaptive behaviour (basic everyday skills). There have been numerous attempts to explain learning disability from the perspectives of education (the ability to use services designed for the 'ordinary' person); psychology (with IQ scores delineating levels of ability/disability); and health and social care (where disability is related to levels of dependency and thus the need for services).

However, like many so-called definitions, these rarely tell the whole story. The learning disabled population is no more a homogenous group than the non-learning disabled population. Some people with a learning disability have accompanying physical deficits, whereas others have none. Some have deficits that affect their ability to understand new information, whereas others will have fewer difficulties in this area, but will struggle to express their understanding. For those who experience autistic spectrum disorders, such as Asperger's Syndrome, their level of intellectual ability may be relatively high, but their social and relational abilities are impaired. The way they experience the world will be very different from the way a non-disabled person experiences it.

Of course, some people with learning disabilities may experience a combination of some or all of these things; their health needs fluctuate with more frequency than the 'ordinary' population, and high levels of medications have a part to play in both their conceptual and performative abilities. All these factors make it very difficult to place a neat label on the life of a person with a 'learning disability' and to feel confident that it describes their experience.

Nature versus nurture

For the social worker, fundamental importance is placed on the influence of environment in the development of all aspects of a person. This perspective is important in the consideration of this client group. Social science research reports extensively on the importance of the child's early experience in bonding with its primary caretaker, and on its need for consistent 'good enough' parenting for the development of physical ability. This is perhaps best demonstrated in 'failure to thrive' studies in which neglected children deteriorate physically, some even fatally, despite having no apparent physical illness. Research also shows the impact of emotional and physical deprivation on intellectual and emotional growth (Kaplan and Sadock, 1994).

The birth of a learning-disabled child very often creates a disruptive crisis in a family for which they were unprepared. When the parents are able to adapt to and manage this crisis at an early stage, they will bond with, nourish and cherish their child (even if, perhaps, still mourning the loss of the 'perfect' child). When the parents are 'stuck' in their grief, or emotionally unable to meet the needs of their child, they will be less able to bond with the baby. This may have a detrimental effect on the baby's physical and mental development, irrespective of the existing disabilities. This can be further complicated by physical difficulties, such as when a child has a limited sucking reflex and finds it difficult to breastfeed, thereby losing a valuable bonding opportunity; or when a disabled child needs specialist care, thereby undergoing a higher level of separation than would normally be expected at such an early stage of life.

Thus, the disruption that a diagnosis of learning disability potentially brings may have repercussions for the physical, emotional and intellectual development of the child, which are indistinguishable from organic factors. John Le Vanier, founder of the L'Arche communities, describes the potential impact on the child's self-understanding:

It is a terrible thing for a child to feel that it has let its parents down and is the cause of their pain and their tears. The wounded heart of the parents wounds the heart of the child... Sometimes I am asked: 'Is a child or adult who has severe mental handicap aware of his or her condition? Do they suffer from this?' For the most part, I don't know. But this I do know: the tiniest infant senses if it is loved and wanted, or not. Similarly, people with a mental handicap, even a severe one, sense immediately whether they are loved and welcomed... If the little one does not sense its mother's love — which not only rejoices in her baby's beauty and uniqueness, but also in its potential for growth, for autonomy and eventual separation from her — the baby feels lost and enters into anguish. It experiences an inner emptiness or an inner suffocation.

(Le Vanier in Ainsworth-Smith and Speck, 1982)

Incidence of learning disability

At present, the learning-disabled community accounts for 3% of the total UK population. This number is increasing annually, despite screening, at a rate of about 1.1% of its total. This increase is due primarily to improved health care and consequent increased longevity. Figures for the incidence in different geographical locations in the UK vary in their accuracy because several regions have not until recently collated figures, owing to the obvious fear of stigma. However, the inaccuracy of information in particular regions has made it difficult to plan and target services effectively, so there is now a move to be more precise in the recording of such information, with Scotland making clear strides forward (Scottish Executive, 2000, 2003).

The changing life-contexts of people with learning disabilities

The last twenty to thirty years have seen a number of changes in the lives of people with learning disabilities. Their increased longevity has been a mixed blessing. In 1939, the average age of mortality for someone with learning disabilities was twelve; now, those who live beyond early adulthood can expect a near-normal lifespan. Although this is a huge improvement, it has also brought with it an increase in illnesses associated with ageing, most notably cancer.

The Down syndrome population has been most affected by increased lifespan. As their age of mortality has increased, so has our understanding that people with this chromosomal abnormality are predisposed to early-onset dementia. The levels are extremely high. In this population, 80% of people can be expected to live into their fifties, but in those over the age of forty there is a 70% or higher incidence of such dementia (Foundation for People with Learning Disabilities, 2001). It is also understood now that people with Down syndrome undergo an accelerated ageing process, thereby encountering chronic medical conditions prematurely; women with Down syndrome, for example, experience menopausal conditions at a much younger age than the ordinary population (McCarthy, 2003).

Although the majority of people with learning disabilities have always lived within their family homes, one of the major changes that they have experienced has been the move away from institutional care. Government legislation throughout Britain will result in the closure of all long-stay learning-disability hospitals by 2006 (Department of Health [DoH], 2001b). This is in keeping with a philosophy of care that demands that people with learning disabilities should not have to access 'segregated' specialist services, but should be able to access mainstream services. Thus, people should not live in healthcare services unless they have physical healthcare needs, and mainstream services are required to adapt to the needs of all users, including those with learning disabilities.

In England, the White Paper *Valuing People* (DoH, 2001b) and, in Scotland, the Scottish Executive Paper *Same as You* (Scottish Executive, 2000) have devised clear action plans for such integration with Government-funded Implementation Teams throughout the countries. In addition, there has been the creation of a new post — that of Healthcare Facilitator (in Scotland, Local Area Coordinator). This professional has a role, as part of a community-based team, to ensure that people with learning disabilities access the same healthcare opportunities as people without disabilities.

Health and learning disability

Over a number of years, healthcare policy has tried to address the inequalities of access that people with a learning disability routinely face (DoH, 1995, 1998). Some of the goals of such policies, even today, are remarkably low-level — such as the goal that every person with a learning disability should be registered with a GP by 2004 (DoH, 2001b).

Despite such goals, we know that the general health of people with learning disabilities is still much poorer than that of the ordinary population. Some of their health concerns are related to the cause of their intellectual disability — for instance, cerebral palsy or heart conditions in people with Down syndrome. However, research has shown that even when the health concern is that experienced by the general population (eg. deficits of sight or hearing), it is much less likely to be diagnosed in people with learning disabilities. People in this community are likely to have five times as many health problems as people in the general population, but are much less likely to visit their GP (DoH, 2001b).

Why then do those people with learning disabilities who visit their GP still fail to have their conditions appropriately diagnosed? The research would suggest that there are at least two reasons: the impact of differential diagnosis and diagnostic overshadowing.

In the former, the healthcare professional fails to make a differentiation between the 'possible diagnostic options within a range of conditions or diseases' (Brown in Scottish Human Services Trust, 2003). This may be related to the limited contact that GPs have with people with learning disabilities and a lack of training concerning this client group. The GP is therefore unable to make distinctions between different types of learning disabilities and associated syndromes, which would enable him to facilitate the best treatment.

Anecdotally, it seems that diagnostic overshadowing is also very common. This occurs when an over-attribution of the learning disability leads the healthcare professional to assume that everything that is presented is a result of the learning disability, as opposed to common physical illnesses. Many carers report that they have been told, 'They have a learning disability, so you have to expect this'. The implications are extremely serious and might account for the late diagnoses of malignancies that are beyond curative treatment.

The situation is exacerbated by at least two further factors. The first is that many people live in social care settings where the care staff have been, until relatively recently, predominantly unqualified. Thus, staff have no background training that would enable them to ascertain early signs of serious ill health. Second, people with learning disabilities often express pain and distress behaviourally rather than verbally. Depending on their ability to conceptualise and understand their own bodies, clients may not be able to convey that they have pain at all, let alone detail its severity and location. Some behavioural communication is fairly clear and straightforward, allowing carers to determine accurately that their client is suggesting physical distress. However, depending on the level of disability, and previous experience of illness, the communication may be made by means of very idiosyncratic behavioural signs. The correct interpretation of the behaviour is therefore crucial; often, learning-disability staff struggle both to interpret the behaviour accurately and to convey their interpretation to health practitioners who do not know the particular client and who may have little experience of working with learning-disabled people.

These problems can be exacerbated by an over-zealous application of the social model of disability, which asserts that people are merely 'differently abled' and which almost rejects medical intervention entirely. Although the medical model has certainly been oppressive towards people with disabilities (consigning them to the category of 'needing to be put right'), there has, at times, been such a swing in the opposite direction as 'to throw the baby out with the bath-water'. This 'swing' crystallises in the social carers' assertion of the primacy of the client's rights over a medical or nursing 'duty of care'. Research by Brown, Burns and Flynn (2003) gives shocking case-study evidence in detailing the case of a learning-disabled woman who had a fungating breast cancer which went untreated until part of her breast actually fell off.

Differential disease profile

As well as being much poorer than in the ordinary population, the health profile of people with learning disabilities is also much more complex. It has a 'layering' of physical and congenital conditions, complications arising from these (eg. epilepsy and degenerative mobility problems), as well as those conditions that arise from predisposing factors and general ageing. Meeting the ongoing needs of this client group is therefore potentially complex, especially with conditions that give rise to palliative care needs. A person with Down syndrome is, for instance, six times more likely to die than an 'ordinary' person, but this is rarely from a malignancy and more likely to be from epilepsy, diabetes or early-onset dementia. In fact, in the learning-disability population generally, the most common causes of deaths are from respiratory and cardiac conditions.

Of course, until now, palliative and hospice care have been cancer-driven, with services effectively targeted at patients with a definable disease progression (House of Commons, 2004: 29). Patients with chronic progressive diseases have accessed palliative care less frequently; consequently, the level of expertise in controlling the symptoms of such conditions is less developed (Higginson, 1997), which has a particular relevance for the palliative care of people with learning disabilities.

Preliminary research indicates that the disease profile of people with learning disabilities may be significantly different from that of the general population when it comes to incidences of cancer (Hogg, Turnbull and Northfield, 2001). This is an area that requires further research, as the comparisons are fairly complex. Although the lifespan of those with learning disabilities has increased, they still have a reduced lifespan, which makes it hard to compare predisposition to cancers, which are still predominantly diseases of old age. Other factors such as comparison of lifestyles or the fact that some physical conditions that give rise to learning disability also give rise to malignancy (eg. tuberous sclerosis) complicate the issue.

However, present research is suggestive of both lower incidences of cancer and a different cancer profile for this client group. Hogg, Northfield and Turnbull (2001) carried out research commissioned by the DoH, which found that only 13% of their sample experienced cancer, as opposed to 26% of the general public. In addition, there was a lower incidence among the learning-disabled of cancers of the bronchus, prostate and breast. By contrast, there was a greatly increased incidence of gastric cancers, which accounted for 58% of learning disability cancer deaths, but only 25% of those cancer sufferers in the general public. The explanation offered for this variance is the much higher infection rate of the bacterial infection *H pylori* in the learning-disabled population (this bacteria has been implicated both in gastric cancers and lymphomas). This research also indicates that there may be significant differences in disease profile in people with Down syndrome. It was found that women with Down syndrome rarely suffered breast cancer, which is suggestive of genetic components. However, it was found that this group is more likely to suffer lymphomas and have a hugely increased risk (10–30%) of childhood leukaemias.

Research of those conditions (including the early dementias) experienced by people with a learning disability suggests that there are pain and symptom-control issues associated with these that are as complicated as those associated with cancers; but, unlike cancer care, the expertise is more limited, the specialist services more sparse, and the coordination of care virtually non-existent (Brown, Burns and Flynn, 2003).

Specialist palliative care social work

The late Frances Sheldon, in her seminal book *Psychosocial Palliative Care* (1997), suggested that there are four underpinning concepts in psychosocial palliative care:

- attachment
- loss
- meaning
- equity.

These concepts serve well in defining the key tasks for the palliative care social worker seeking to provide appropriate services to people with learning disabilities, and those that matter to them.

Equity

The issue of equity is fundamental for this client group, with a highly disproportionate number of those with mild learning disabilities being found in Social Class V (Sinason, 1992). Framed in legislative responses is a recognition of the inequity that many people with learning disabilities encounter in daily life (DoH, 2000, 2001b). Unfortunately, this is clearly the case in cancer and palliative care services too.

For reasons already discussed, people with learning disabilities who have cancer are likely to be diagnosed late (as in David's case). An additional reason for late diagnoses is the lack of access such people have to screening services, which was the subject of a 1998 Mencap study. Of the ordinary population of women who were eligible for cervical screening, 85% accessed this service. Of the eligible learning-disabled population, only a maximum of 17% did so, and this fell dramatically to 3% of those people living at home. Breast screening figures were rather better: in comparison to 76% of the ordinary population, 50% of the female learning-disabled population (who eligible to do so) accessed screening, which fell to 17% of those people living at home. However, when offered breast screening, more than 90% of women with learning disabilities took up this offer, undermining the idea that there may be apathy about health in this group.

When diagnosed with a malignancy, it is not uncommon for a person with learning disabilities to be offered less 'heroic' (ie. difficult) treatments than the general public. There are several reasons for this: there may be assumptions made about the ability of the person to withstand difficult treatments, for example, or issues of whether the person is able to consent to them. However, assumptions about quality of life often become clinical judgements about the value of life, and this can impair the clinician's ability to be objective in deciding treatment options (Wolfensberger, 1987).

It is to be hoped that the UK National Cancer Plan and the formalising of patient care pathways, specific to disease type, will minimise subjective treatment decisions (DoH, 2000b). It is also hoped that Healthcare Facilitators and Local Area Coordinators will be able to effect this process. However, given that these are likely to be mainly social care professionals with no medical or nursing training, there will continue to be a vital role for the palliative care social worker in the multiplicity of settings in which they work.

Of course, the palliative care social worker does not have medical or nursing training either, but will have developed a wealth of experience in the palliative care context, attuning their sensitivity to issues of inequity of treatment. The role requires daily involvement in enabling the psychosocial aspects of care to be given their appropriate level of priority, and they are thus experienced in advocating for and facilitating the advocacy skills of patients and their families within a medical context.

Case study: Geraldine's story

When Geraldine was diagnosed with cancer, it was during emergency surgery that had been carried out without her explicit consent on the basis of being in her 'best interest'. When she was recovering from surgery, a limited explanation of her condition was given to her but did not include the diagnosis of cancer. As her condition progressed, a difference of perspective between the professional learning-disability carers and Geraldine's family developed.

Staff felt that it was Geraldine's 'right' to know about her cancer and that she would die from it. The family felt that the news would be too difficult for Geraldine; that she would not cope with it and should not be told because it would hasten her death and lead to her dying in a distressed state.

The palliative care social worker's role was to advocate for Geraldine that it was her right to know what 'she' wanted to know.

The skill of advocacy is tested to its limit in such situations, but social work's valuing of autonomy and choice (advocated by palliative care) demands that if no other team member is willing to take on such a challenge, then the social worker is duty bound to do so. Sometimes, this duty will be fulfilled by asking questions within the multidisciplinary team; sometimes it will be by enabling formal and informal carers to explore and formulate their own challenging questions; sometimes it will be by enabling the person with a learning disability to communicate their wish for active treatment if they are able to understand the consequences of it. However it is done, it is the duty of the social worker to convey to the individual their unique value so that they feel they are important enough to demand what is their right.

The importance of this duty cannot be underestimated with this client group, many of whom have been told explicitly and implicitly throughout their lives that they should not exist — that they are a drain on their family and on society's resources (Sinason, 1995). Against a backdrop of such express and subliminal messages, it can be extremely hard for this person to feel that they have an innate right to an equality of treatment to their non-disabled peers. Much more subject to the opinions of others, and especially those in medical settings, the client may need a great deal of support to take on the daunting task of challenging those in power. The social worker, with their training in anti-oppressive practice, is well-placed to undertake an empowering partnership role with the client.

This is, of course, still the case when the client makes an informed choice not to receive treatment. Although advocacy of the person's rights and choices may be more difficult in this scenario and require much soul-searching as to how competent the client is to make this decision (which will ultimately result in a fatal outcome), the social worker should be willing to take on this role, irrespective of their own beliefs and values.

Meaning

The longer one works within palliative care, the more clearly one sees that 'meaning' is the crux of the quality of the dying experience, both for the patient and those who love and are loved by them. This is a multi-faceted concept and includes the sense one makes of the illness and how one decides to deal with it — ie. whether to fight it, reject it, or accept it. It is also at the heart of those 'not so good' deaths in which resolution is not achieved and death is therefore even more distressing. It is the lens through which we judge our past and present, and through which we envisage the future.

It is clear from all the research and literature on hope in palliative care that communication is a key building block in the construction of helpful meanings. Bad news, badly told, psychologically disorders the patient and robs them of hope, disabling them from finding resourceful ways of approaching their challenging situation. By contrast, constructive, positive support from professionals, family and other patients not only improves the quality of life of the patient, but may also positively affect their prognosis (Spiegel, 1989).

Within this section, we will think about some of the practical issues related to communication, especially within breaking the news of the diagnosis and in gaining informed consent. We shall also consider issues related to life review and the related spiritual aspects. Throughout this section, the emphasis is on the palliative care social worker's role in improving the patient's quality of life.

Communication

Palliative care prides itself in having led the way in enlightening medical staff to the importance of sensitive communication. Within a few decades, doctors have moved away from the opinion that patients should not be told of their diagnosis if it is cancer (believing that this would hasten their death) to a consensus that everyone should be told (Oken, Billings, Maynard in Buckman,

1992). However, the emphasis has rightly progressed from 'whether' someone should be told to 'how' they should be told, with a number of patients and families telling detailed stories of the negative impact of being told 'the truth, the whole truth, and nothing but the truth'.

Research shows that how the news is broken is crucial to how the patient is able to deal with the diagnosis and make decisions about the treatment. Handled too bluntly, the patient may be robbed of hope and not see the point of complying with the treatment; told too subtly, on the other hand, they may not understand the significance of the news in a way that enables them to make the life changes and decisions necessary (Maguire and Faulkener, 1988).

Such communication is a highly complex skill and in the UK this is acknowledged in the provision of 'advanced communication skills training' for all senior-level oncology staff. It is further endorsed in the UK National Institute for Clinical Excellence (NICE) guidelines for supportive and specialist palliative care (NHS, 2004). A six-step communication model has been developed and is being used to good effect throughout the UK.

However, although legislation pays lip service to the idea that the model should be adapted to the needs of those with sensory or intellectual disabilities, there are presently no guidelines for how this should be done (NHS, 2004). This fact, coupled with the lack of input regarding learning disability in general medical and nursing training, means that people with learning disabilities are desperately disadvantaged when confronted in a consultation with a generally trained health professional. This application of the traditional medical model of service delivery effectively disenfranchises the learning-disabled patient from any possibility of a partnership with their medical team, and renders them powerless in the resulting dynamic.

Furthermore, in a recent (unpublished) piece of small-scale research, McEnhill (2004) found that in interviews with ten learning-disabled people who had received bad news about their own terminal illness or that of a close family member, not one had received this news from a member of the medical team. Thus, anecdotally at least, it would appear that people with learning disabilities are often not told about their illnesses by medical staff, with their carers being left with the dilemmas of whether and how to do so. Since communication is a two-way process, the relevant oncologists are unable to gain the necessary sense of what is important to the patient before offering a range of treatment options. In Geraldine's case she was considered to be 'not compliant with treatment' but in actual fact her diagnosis, prognosis and treatment options had never been discussed with her by any member of her medical or nursing team.

Consent to treatment is a thorny issue when working with people with learning disabilities and, again anecdotally, it would appear that many medics assume that because a person has a cognitive deficit, they are unable to consent to treatment. Sadly, some then go on to assert that it is not possible to treat the patient without such informed consent. Recent legislation in Scotland (The Mental Incapacity Act Scotland, Scottish Executive, 2000b) has brought clarity to the situation, as will the Mental Capacity Bill in England, if enacted.

Consistent application of this legislation by general medical staff may take longer to achieve.

Within the confines of this chapter it is not possible to discuss alternative approaches in detail, but some guidelines may be useful to bear in mind:

Guidelines for communicating with someone with a learning disability

⌘ It is useful, as a starting point, to explore a developmental psychology model in communicating with someone with a learning disability — ie. in addition to their chronological age, consider their developmental age. What are the challenges of communicating with someone at this developmental stage? Are they, for instance, able to think abstractly or do they apply an over-literal explanation to information given? An example from children's literature is where a child understood that a 'dye injection' was a 'die injection' and was understandably very scared of the procedure (Myerscough and Ford, 1989).

⌘ In addition, remember that people with learning disabilities do not always link concepts in the way that we expect them to, so that someone may not know that serious illness can lead to death. Confirm the meaning of what, to you, might seem clear or obvious.

⌘ People with learning disabilities, like all of us, learn from experience so check what their previous experience of illness and death is. From this, they may have been able to link concepts such as illness and dying, which they had not been able to before.

⌘ Some 'breaking-bad-news' models for the general population (eg. Maguire) suggest using 'hierarchies of euphemisms' to communicate. In working with a person with a learning disability, however, avoid the use of euphemisms and remember that a too-subtle approach (eg. the use of warning shots or expecting the person to ask questions) may only create confusion.

⌘ Try always to supplement words with pictorial information and consistently check with the person with learning disabilities and their carer that what is being said is understood.

⌘ Remember that the person may not have a good understanding of the passage of time. This is extremely important when trying to convey information about prognosis and should inform the decision as to when the person should be told, if ever, that their condition is terminal.

In addition, there are some useful things to remember when dealing with consent and people with learning disabilities:

- ⌘ Everyone should be presumed to be competent unless proven otherwise (ie. not presumed to be incompetent).
- ⌘ People are not universally competent (ie. it is possible to be competent to consent to the removal of a painful decayed tooth whilst perhaps not being competent to consent to palliative chemotherapy).
- ⌘ No-one can consent to treatment on behalf of another adult (incapacitated or not).
- ⌘ Incapacity in and of itself is not grounds for refusing to give medical treatment; doctors are required to act in the 'best interests' of a patient, irrespective of their ability to consent.
- ⌘ One must always check that the full implications of accepting or refusing a treatment are understood. For instance, Mary refused an operation to remove her breast cancer because she was frightened of operations, but it was many months before she began to suspect that the cancer, if not removed, could kill her.

Life review

Scottish poet Robert Burns reminds us in his poem 'To a Mouse' that humans, as far as we know, are unique in their ability to experience regret for the past and dread for the future:

> *Still thou are blest, compared wi me, The present only toucheth thee,*
> *But Och! I backward cast my e'e On prospects drear!*
> *An forward, tho I canna see, I guess and fear!*

Robert Burns (1759–1796)

These insights present both opportunity and crisis when confronting one's mortality. Hence, it is one of the main tasks of the palliative care professional to facilitate a life review so that the person is able to 'tie up loose ends' and find acceptable meanings for the events of their life. This task carries on into the bereavement care of those of significance to the patient.

In working with people with learning disabilities, the palliative care social worker has much to offer in this area of practice. Many people with learning disabilities are unable to detail their life history accurately, and rely heavily on the storytellers. When these are family members, the social worker is able to bring the family together and facilitate some shared identity work. Sadly, if the person has spent most of his or her life in institutional care, there is likely to be little that details the unique context of this person's life, as opposed to all the other service users within that service.

The task, then, for the social worker is to create a sense of context with and for this person. Some of this may be very simple and expressed in a concrete tool, such as a life-story book that details the person's likes and dislikes, schools, previous homes, etc (McEnhill, 2000). Some of it may be incredibly painful and the worker will require good supervision to enable them to stay with the pain of multiple losses (Sinason, 1995). For many, the sense of identity may have been developed with a concentration on disability rather than ability, and will require reframing. Equally, if they are aware of what Sinason and Wolfensberger (1987) call society's 'death wish' towards them, this will have a unique influence on how they understand their last days.

It will be crucial for the worker in this scenario to be committed to the fact that the most important thing about the person is the uniqueness of their story and not their disability, which is just one element of the story. They will need to be creative in finding ways to express the story for the patient and for others with whom they want to share it. Given the extremely high levels and variety of abuse experienced by people with learning disabilities, workers will need to be able to suspend their judgement and hear how things have 'really' been for this person throughout their life.

In summary, there are several important points to bear in mind when helping a learning-disabled person with a life review:

⌘ There are lessons to be learned from reminiscence therapy because the story may be held intact within the individual, but without the correct cues or questions it may not be uncovered.

⌘ The person's own interpretation of events is as important as any 'factual' information.

⌘ The questions that normally have to be resolved for those who are terminally ill are 'Who am I?' and 'What has my life been about?' and implicitly 'How do I want to be mourned and remembered?' For the person with a learning disability, they may additionally want to be assured that they will be remembered; the life review, if captured in a life storybook, can be evidence of this.

⌘ It is important to detail achievements.

⌘ It is important to record relationships and what the person has meant to those around them, with some quotations if possible.

⌘ Not everything in the life review needs be hugely significant; it is the uniqueness of the story, not its drama, which is important.

Spirituality

In the context of meaning, a final word needs to be said about spirituality. Spirituality is often described as having to do with questions of ultimate meaning. Sadly, there is little spiritual care provision for people with learning disabilities, whether they have a faith or not. This lack seems to be something of a taboo in secular care services because many staff fear that their clients may be indoctrinated into religious beliefs that have previously disenfranchised them (eg. the belief that learning disability is the result of personal sin).

However, in the field of palliative care, spiritual care is seen as a core service and vital for people coming to terms with the end of their life. Whilst the palliative care social worker may not feel they can provide spiritual care, they should advocate that people with learning disabilities are likely to have the same range of spiritual needs as everyone else, and encourage carers to think about how these may best be met. For some, this will have a religious expression; for others, it will be through, say, pictures of nature or listening to music.

How spiritual needs and beliefs are expressed will vary from person to person. Work by Professor John Swinton for the Foundation for People with Learning Disabilities is a useful resource in expanding one's appreciation of this area of care (Swinton, 1999, 2001, 2004).

Attachment and loss

Given that attachment and loss are inseparable, they will be discussed in the same section. Attachment is a concept developed initially by John Bowlby (1969) and reformulated several times by a number of theorists from various perspectives. Attachment describes the human drive to relate and the need to develop close bonds with primary caregivers (Bowlby, 1969; Rutter, 1972). There are many different explanations as to the source of the drive and the reasons for it, the most plausible being related to survival (Cooper and Roth, 2002). Whilst there are varying perspectives on the influence of the environment on individuals, almost all people would see the early bonding experience of children, which results in attachment behaviour, to be hugely significant. In fact, some definitions of mental illness define the inability to bond (by the age of two years) as a symptom of psychopathology.

One of the most amazing aspects of working with people with learning disabilities is the prevalent belief, in a number of settings, that they do not attach and that others do not attach to them in the same way as in the ordinary population. This may be explicit or implicit, but common examples are:

⌘   Parents being told to leave their disabled baby behind in hospital, to go home, forget them and start again.
⌘   Services having little records of the person within the context of their family; for example, whether they are the first or third child.

- ⌘ Parents being expected to view the untimely death of their learning-disabled child as a 'blessed release'.
- ⌘ People not expecting someone to grieve the separation or death of a close family member or friend.
- ⌘ People suggesting that so long as the physical care needs are met, the person with a learning disability will not experience the distress of separation. Or, to put it another way, any carer is as good as another to the person with a learning disability as long as they take good care of the primary physical care needs.

If one cannot attach, one cannot experience loss. Given the common assumption that learning-disabled people do not form attachments, it is perhaps unsurprising that people in the ordinary population often assume that learning-disabled people do not grieve, which has the knock-on effect that their grief goes neglected or even unrecognised.

Only recently have people started to accept that people with learning disabilities may grieve and may need support during their bereavement. Despite a number of articles on the subject, and training sessions throughout the country, it is still fairly common to find that care staff do not acknowledge the loss in the way they would with their 'ordinary' peers (Hollins and Esterhausen, 1997). Sadly, this results in bereaved people with learning disabilities developing depression and self-injurious and challenging behaviours as the only means of expressing their distress. Research by Emerson (1977) suggests that the bereaved person with a learning disability is more likely to receive a behaviour-modification programme than counselling.

Palliative care social workers have not always promoted the case of these bereaved people. Some small-scale research has shown that palliative care social workers rarely offer bereavement counselling to learning-disabled clients and that many thought those clients should be referred onto a specialist agency (Bowd, 1998).

However, there are at least two problems with this perspective. First, there are very few specialist bereavement services specifically for people with learning disabilities. Second, to suggest that specialist help is required is to pathologise the grief and to indulge in a psychosocial over-attribution of the learning disability such as would not be applied to any other client group.

There is no doubt that the bereavement care of learning-disabled people may be complex due to the number of losses they are likely to have experienced; the high level of unresolved losses; and the fact that they may have had their access to rites of passage and healthy expression of grief obstructed. In addition, some of the cognitive deficits may stretch the skills of the bereavement helper, though arguably no more so than in the bereavement care of children, of those with a mental illness, or of those whose first language is not English. We would rightly want to advocate the right to good bereavement care for all of these groups.

It is the role of the palliative care social worker to assert that even those with profound learning disabilities will have some ability to attach to their primary caregivers and to experience separation from them as loss. Only those with a mental age of less than seven months may potentially be regarded as having little capacity to experience the separation as loss (having not by this stage reached the ability to experience object constancy). However, even in these cases, it is often clear that they recognise those with whom they have a familial relationship, compared with those who are only their temporary carers. Thus, not to respond to their loss-initiated distress is a failure of care.

In terms of bereavement counselling techniques, a great deal can be learned from developmental perspectives and thus from child-bereavement practitioners. Irrespective of this, the overarching principles are the same — eg. listen to the client, and move at his or her pace, because how they define and experience the loss will be unique to them and should be responded to as such. For those who suggest that a more complex psychoanalytic approach cannot be undertaken with these clients, the seminal work of Sinason (1995) and the more recent but formative work of Blackman (2000, 2003) should inform their practice.

Conclusion

Palliative care social work with people with learning disabilities presents us with unique opportunities to challenge and develop our skills. The values of palliative care enacted in our practice have the potential to enable the learning-disabled client to gain a new reflection of themselves and, despite dying or grieving, to experience growth and achievement. Although it may stretch our abilities, it requires, in the main, a revisiting of primary social work skills and values. Above all, it requires a reaffirmation of the importance of relationship and use of self. When we get it wrong, these clients, having learned to expect so little, are among the most forgiving. When we get it right, we will find that it is not at all difficult to assure the client that their life has mattered and that they will be mourned and remembered in years to come.

References

Ainsworth-Smith I, Speck P (1982) *Letting Go: Caring for the Dying and Bereaved.* SPCK, London

Bambang S, Spencer NJ, Logan S, Gill L (2000) Cause-specific perinatal death rates, birth weight and deprivation in the West Midlands, 1991-93. *Child Care Health Dev* **26**(1): 73–82

Blackman N (2003) *Loss and Learning Disability*. Worth Publishing Ltd, London

Blackman N (ed) (2000) *Living with Loss: Helping People with Learning Disabilities Cope with Bereavement and Loss*. Pavilion Publishing, Brighton

Bowlby (1969) Attachment. Vol 1 of *Attachment and Loss*. London: Hogarth Press. New York: Basic Books; Harmondsworth: Penguin (1971)

Bowd S (1998) Unpublished dissertation: Meeting the Psychological Needs of People with Learning Disabilities Facing Bereavement: an Exploration of Practice in Palliative Care Settings. Department of Social Work, Middlesex University

Brown H, Burns S, Flynn M (2003) *Dying Matters*. London Salomons Centre Kent & Foundation for People with Learning Disabilities, London

Buckman R (1992) *How to Break Bad News: a Guide for Healthcare Professionals*. Papermac, London

Cooper T, Roth I (2002) *Challenging Psychological Issues*. Open University Press, Milton Keynes

DoH (1995) *The Health of the Nation: a Strategy for People with Learning Disability*. HMSO, London

DoH (1998) *Signposts for Success in Commissioning and Providing Health Services for People with Learning Disabilities*. DoH, Wetherby

DoH (2000) *Good Practice in Breast and Cervical Screening of Women with Learning Disabilities*. DoH, London

DoH (2000b) *The NHS Cancer Plan: a Plan for Investment, a Plan for Reform*. DoH, London

DoH (2001a) *Seeking Consent: Working with People with Learning Disabilities*. DoH, London

DoH (2001b) *Valuing People: a New Strategy for Learning Disability for the 21st Century*. White Paper. DoH, London

Emerson P (1977) Covert grief reactions in mentally retarded clients. *Ment Retard* **15**(6): 45–7

Foundation for People with Learning Disabilities (2001) *Down's Syndrome and Dementia: Briefing for Commissioners*. Mental Health Foundation, London

Heffer RW, Kelley ML (1994) Non-organic failure to thrive: developmental outcomes and psychosocial assessment and intervention issues. *Res Dev Disability* **15**: 247–68

Higginson I (1997) *Palliative and Terminal Care in Health Care Needs Assessment*. Stevens A, Raftery J (eds) Radcliffe, Oxford

Hogg J, Northfield J, Turnbull J (2001) *Cancer and People with Learning Disabilities: the Evidence from Published Studies and Experiences from Cancer Services*. BILD, Kidderminster

Hollins S, Esterhuyzen A (1997) Bereavement and grief in adults with learning disabilities. *Br J Psychiat* **170**: 497–501

House of Commons Health Committee (2004) *Palliative Care 4th Report 2003–2004*. HC454-1, London

Kaplan HI, Sadock BJ, Grebb JA (1994) *Synopsis of Psychiatry*. Williams & Wilkins, USA

Lipe-Godson P, Goebel B. Perception of age and death in mentally retarded adults. *Ment Retard* **21**: 68–75

McCarthy M (2003) *Supporting Women with Learning Disabilities through the Menopause.* Pavilion Publishing, Brighton

McEnhill L (2000) Guided mourning interventions. In: Blackman N (ed) *Living with Loss: Helping People with Learning Disabilities Cope with Bereavement and Loss.* Pavilion Publishing, Brighton

McEvoy J (1989) Investigating the concept of death in adults who are mentally handicapped. *Br J Ment Subnormal* **35**(2): 69

McGrother C, Thorp C, Taub N, Machado O (2001) Prevalence, disability and need in adults with severe learning disabilities. *Tizard Learn Disabil Rev* **6**: 4–13

Maguire P, Faulkner A (1988) How to do it: communicate with cancer patients and their relatives. *BMJ* **297**: 907–24

MENCAP (1998) *The NHS: Health for All? People with Learning Disabilities and Healthcare.* Mencap National Centre, London

Myerscough PR, Ford F (1989) *Talking with Patients: Keys to Good Communication.* 3rd edn. Oxford University Press, Oxford

NHS (2004) *Guidance on Cancer Services: Improving Supportive and Palliative Care for Adults with Cancer — The Manual.* NICE, London

Oswin M (1991) *Am I Allowed to Cry?* Souvenir Press Ltd, London

Russell O, Stanley M (1996) *A Literature Review of Local Variation in the Needs of People with Learning Disabilities for Health Service Input.* Bristol: Norah Fry Research Centre, University of Bristol

Rutter M (1972) *Maternal Deprivation Reassessed.* Harmondsworth, Penguin

Scottish Executive (2000) *The Same as You: Review of Services for People with Learning Disabilities.* Scottish Executive, Scotland

Scottish Executive (2000b) *The Adults with Incapacity Act.* Scottish Executive, Scotland

Scottish Executive (2003) Statistics Release: Adults with Learning Disabilities Implementation of 'The Same as You?'. www.scotland.gov.uk/stats/bulletin/00326.pdf

Scottish Human Services Trust (2003) *Palliative Care and People with Learning Disabilities.* SHS Trust Edinburgh

Sheldon F (1997) *Psychosocial Palliative Care: Good Practice in the Care of the Dying and Bereaved.* Thornes (Publishers) Ltd, Cheltenham

Sinason V (1992) *Mental Handicap and the Human Condition: New Approaches from the Tavistock.* Free Association Books Ltd, London

Spiegel D, Bloom JR, Kraemer HC, *et al* (1989) Effect of psychosocial treatment on survival of patients with metastatic breast cancer. *Lancet* **2**: 888–91

Swinton J (1999) *Building a Church for Strangers: Theology, Church and Learning Disabilities.* Contact Pastoral Trust, Edinburgh

Swinton J (2001) *A Space to Listen: Meeting the Spiritual Needs of People with Learning Disabilities.* The Mental Health Foundation, London

Swinton J, Powrie E (2004) *Why Are We Here: Meeting the Spiritual Needs of People with Learning Disabilities.* The FPLD Mental Health Foundation, London

Tuffrey-Wijne I (2003) The palliative care needs of people with intellectual disabilities: a literature review. *Palliat Med* **17**(8): 55–62

Winnicott DW (1989: reprint) *The Family and Individual Development*. Routledge, London/New York

Wolfensberger W (1987) *The New Genocide of Handicapped and Afflicted People*. Syracuse University Division of Special Education and Rehabilitation, Syracuse

Index

A

acceptance 42, 70, 92, 105, 106, 121, 127, 138
activities of daily living (ADLs) 136
Alzheimer's disease 131, 141, 144
anticipatory grief 141
Asperger's syndrome 146
assessment 3, 4, 15, 17, 35, 64, 85, 86, 88, 91, 98, 100, 124, 125, 128, 136–138, 162
attachment 67, 69, 98, 151, 159

B

Bangladeshis 39
bereavement vii, viii, 1, 3, 5, 10–18, 22, 24, 28, 36, 57–91, 96, 99, 121, 126, 130, 132, 135, 140–142, 157, 160
Bereavement Service Coordinators 83
best fit 55, 57
black Caribbeans 39
blood relatives 90
body language 93, 101, 138

C

care management 30, 32, 137
closure 78, 104, 105, 107, 114, 148
Commission for Racial Equality (CRW) 38
confidentiality 23, 60, 61, 138
consistency 7, 33, 58, 60
continuity theories 69
coping styles 69, 73, 74

Certificate of Qualification in Social Work (CQSW) 5
cultural competence 42

D

degree in social work 7, 14
dementia 65, 102, 131–144, 148, 150
DipSW 6, 7, 13, 17
Discharge Planning Meetings (DPM) 54
Down's syndrome 148–151
drama 113, 158
dramatherapy 115

E

ecomaps 97
emotional work 44
end vii, 10, 18, 38, 40, 59, 61, 71, 78, 83, 104, 105, 107, 111, 114, 120, 123, 132, 134, 139, 141, 143, 158
ending 104–114
England 5, 7, 8, 9, 18, 21, 39, 43, 50, 104, 115, 134, 148, 155
equity 151, 152
euthanasia 16, 139, 140

F

Family Support Team 99

G

God 2, 24, 70, 116, 117, 120–122
good communication 82, 125
good endings 105